Edited by E.I. Hernández-Jiménez, E.M. Rakhanskaya

ROSACEA AND COUPEROSIS
IN COSMETIC DERMATOLOGY & SKINCARE PRACTICE

Cosmetics & Medicine
Publishing

Author/Editor:
Elena I. Hernández-Jiménez, *Ph.D.*

Editor:
Ekaterina M. Rakhanskaya, *M.D.* Neurologist, radiation safety specialist

Contributors:
Vera I. Albanova, *M.D., Ph.D., Prof.* Dermatologist
Natalya G. Kalashnikova, *M.D.* Surgeon, dermatologist, laser therapist
Diana S. Urakova, *M.D., Ph.D.* Dermatologist, laser therapist

ROSACEA AND COUPEROSIS IN COSMETIC DERMATOLOGY AND SKINCARE PRACTICE

Rosacea on average affects 5% of all people on Earth, and couperosis — a problem for a considerable number of fair-skinned people that catches up with them, if not in their youth, then as they age — is one of the symptoms of photoaging. Therefore, any specialist working with skin cannot avoid "encountering" these conditions.

However, even though rosacea was regarded exclusively as a dermatological problem for a long time, and couperosis was deemed virtually impossible to cope with, modern research and developments in the field of dermatology give specialists a variety of working tools to correct these unpleasant aesthetic defects.

The specialty of our book is that we look at cosmetic approaches that can help patients with rosacea and couperosis. We not only vouch that these approaches work but know from experience that cosmetic care can slow down the progression of these diseases. Thus, it not only saves patients from aggressive dermatologic treatment but also significantly improves their quality of life.

This publication will detail the current understanding of the etiology and pathogenesis of rosacea. We consider these facts important to know because recent research has dramatically changed the primary image of the disease and the treatment approaches. We now understand that what used to be considered a cure by dermatologists may sometimes worsen the skin condition of rosacea patients. We will thus examine in detail how to build a primary therapy based on these modern findings, what methods and products can be used, and what should be excluded from therapy and care programs offered to patients with rosacea.

The same applies to couperosis, as we will once again explain this condition and how it differs from rosacea, allowing specialists to apply the most effective therapy, particularly laser treatment. How do these methods work? How to prepare and protect the skin? Whether there is an effect from topical and injectable methods (and what kind of effect)? All these questions are discussed in detail in the relevant sections.

This book is a must-read for all specialists in aesthetic medicine, students pursuing degrees in dermatological specialties, and even patients who want to effectively resolve the problems of rosacea and couperosis.

ISBN 978-1-970196-22-1 (paperback)
ISBN 978-1-970196-08-5 (eBook – Adobe PDF)
ISBN 978-1-970196-16-0 (eBook – ePUB)

© Cosmetics & Medicine Publishing LLC, 2024
© Cover photo: Cast Of Thousands / Shutterstock

FirstEditing

English version is edited and certified by the FirstEditing.Com, Inc. (USA).

Author/Editor

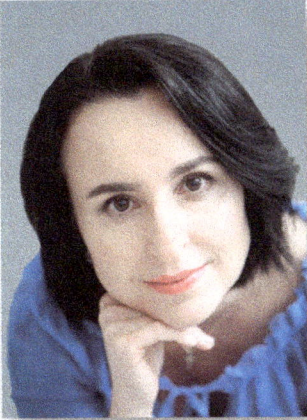

Elena I. Hernández-Jiménez, *Ph.D.*

Biophysicist, scientific journalist

Editor-in-chief of Cosmetics and Medicine Publishing

Chairperson of the Executive Board of the International Society of Applied Corneotherapy (I.A.C.)

Author and co-author of numerous publications in professional magazines, co-author and editor of the book series *Fundamentals of Cosmetic Dermatology & Skincare*, *Cosmetic Dermatology & Skincare Practice*, *Cosmetic Chemistry for Dermatology & Skincare Specialists* and others

Speaker at international conferences, author of training seminars and webinars for professionals in the field of skincare

Professional interests: biology and physiology of the skin, skin permeability, cosmetic chemistry, anti-age medicine, physiotherapy in dermatology and aesthetic medicine, skin analysis and imaging

Table of Contents

List of abbreviations 9

Introduction 10

PART I

ROSACEA

Chapter 1. Etiology and pathogenesis...........................**15**

1.1. Immune factor 15

    1.1.1. IL-17 and T-cell immunity imbalance 17

    1.1.2. Mast cells 18

    1.1.3. Neurovascular dysfunction and neurogenic
        inflammation 20

        Sensory receptors of cells 20

        Neurotransmitters 22

        Genetic predisposition 23

1.2. Skin barrier function 24

1.3. Microbiome 24

    1.3.1. Skin microbiome 24

    1.3.2. Gut microbiome 26

1.4. Genetic predisposition 27

1.5. Rosacea-contributing factors 28

    1.5.1. Triggering factors 28

    1.5.2. Risk factors and comorbidities 31

Chapter 2. Classification and clinical manifestation
    (Albanova V.I.) **33**

2.1. Classification 33

2.2. Clinical picture 36

    2.2.1. General characterization 36

    2.2.2. Clinical manifestation of rosacea according
        to the 2002 classification 36

        Pre-rosacea 37

Erythematotelangiectatic rosacea 38

Papulopustular (inflammatory) rosacea 39

Phymatous rosacea 40

Ophthalmorosacea 41

2.2.3. Clinical manifestation of rosacea according
to the 2017 classification 41

2.2.4. Specific forms of rosacea 44

Rosacea granulomatosa. 44

Rosacea conglobata 44

Rosacea fulminans 44

Rosacea gram-negative 45

Chapter 3. Diagnostics *(Albanova V.I.)* **46**

3.1. Diagnosis 46

3.2. Differential diagnosis 47

3.2.1. Erythematotelangiectatic rosacea 47

3.2.2. Rosacea papulopustulosa. 49

Acne vulgaris. 49

Perioral dermatitis. 51

Demodicosis 51

Chapter 4. Impact of lifestyle on rosacea treatment **53**

Chapter 5. Medication treatment **55**

5.1. Drugs 55

Kallikrein-5 inhibitors. 55

Vasoconstrictor drugs 55

Antibacterial drugs 56

Antiprotozoal and antiparasitic drugs 56

Retinoids. 56

5.2. Recommended administration regimen 56

Chapter 6. Cosmetic care. **59**

6.1. Selecting cosmetic products 59

6.2. Skin cleansing 61

6.2.1. Cleansers 62

6.2.2. Choosing a cleaning product 64

    Normal sebum production. 64

    Low sebum production. 64

    Sebum overproduction (oily skin). 64

6.2.3. Cleansing routine 65

6.2.4. For men: shaving rosacea-affected skin. 66

6.3. Restoring and strengthening the skin barrier 66

6.3.1. Hydrolipid mantle and surface pH 66

6.3.2. Strengthening the lipid barrier 68

6.3.3. Moisturizing the *stratum corneum* 70

6.4. Normalizing the skin microbiome 71

6.5. Special cosmetic ingredients for rosacea 73

6.5.1. Antioxidants 73

6.5.2. Zinc 75

6.5.3. Niacinamide 76

6.5.4. Tranexamic acid. 77

6.5.5. Azelaic acid 78

6.6. Sunscreen products 78

6.7. Decorative cosmetics 83

6.7.1. How to apply makeup to minimize irritation. 83

Chapter 7. Energy-based methods. 85

7.1. Light therapy: mechanism of action 85

7.2. Laser and IPL devices 88

7.3. Treating vascular alterations *(Kalashnikova N.G., Urakova D.S.)* 90

    Pulsed dye laser (PDL). 90

    Potassium-titanium-phosphate laser (KTP) 90

    Neodymium laser (Nd:YAG) 92

    Intense pulsed light (IPL) 92

7.4. Treating connective tissue changes
(Kalashnikova N.G., Urakova D.S.) 92

7.4.1. Dissection of altered anatomical entities 92

7.4.2. Tissue remodeling. 94

7.5. RF microneedling 96

Chapter 8. Botulinum toxin therapy **97**

8.1. Mechanism of action 97

8.2. Clinical experience 98

8.3. Rosacea-like steroid dermatitis 100

Chapter 9. Diet in rosacea. **103**

9.1. Food triggers 103

    Alcohol 103

    Unfermented tea 103

    Caffeine 104

    Niacin-rich food. 104

    Spicy food. 104

    Cinnamaldehyde 105

    Histamine-rich food 105

    Fatty food 105

    Dairy products. 105

9.2. Nutrients indicated for patients with rosacea 106

    9.2.1. Supporting the skin's defense mechanisms 106

    Omega-3 unsaturated fatty acids. 106

    Zinc. 106

    9.2.2. Restoring the balance of the intestinal microbiome. 107

    Prebiotics 107

    Probiotics 107

9.3. Preventing the cardiovascular disorders 108

9.4. General recommendations 109

PART II
COUPEROSIS

Chapter 1. Etiology. **111**

Chapter 2. Clinical manifestation **113**

Chapter 3. Diagnostics **115**

Chapter 4. Treating couperosis **117**

4.1. Lifestyle 117

4.2. Cosmetic care for couperosis 118

    4.2.1 Skin cleansing 118

    4.2.2. Home care 118

    4.2.3. Cosmetic ingredients with vasoconstrictive
        properties 118

    4.2.4. Cosmetic camouflage 119

Chapter 5. Injection treatment **120**

Chapter 6. Energy-based therapy. **121**

6.1. Electrical methods 121

    6.1.1. Microcurrent therapy 121

    6.1.2. Electrocoagulation and RF microneedling. 121

6.2. Light therapy 122

6.3. Cryodestruction 122

Afterwords **124**

References **125**

List of abbreviations

CAMP — cathelicidin antimicrobial peptide

cAMP — cyclic adenosine monophosphate

CGRP — calcitonin gene-related peptide

DNA — deoxyribonucleic acid

Er:glass — erbium:glass laser

Er:YAG — erbium:yttrium-aluminum-garnet crystal laser

Er:YSGG — erbium:yttrium-scandium-gallium-garnet crystal laser

FDA — U.S. Food and Drug Administration

FGF-2 — fibroblast growth factor 2

IL — interleukin

IPL — intense pulsed light

IR — infrared light

KLK — kallikrein

KTP — potassium-titanium-phosphate crystal laser

mRNA — messenger ribonucleic acid

MLE — multi-lamellar emulsions

MMP — matrix metalloproteinase

Nd:YAG — neodymium:yttrium-aluminum-garnet crystal laser

NMF — natural moisturizing factor

NLRP3 — NOD-like receptor protein 3

PACAP — pituitary adenylate cyclase-activating polypeptide

PAR2 — protease-activated transmembrane receptor 2

PABA — para-aminobenzoic acid

PCA — pyrrolidone carboxylic acid

PDL — pulsed dye laser

pH — acidity value (*pondus Hydrogenii*)

RF — radiofrequency

RNA — ribonucleic acid

ROSCO — consensus of the international expert group on rosacea (ROSacea COnsensus)

ROS — reactive oxygen species

SMA — spatially modulated ablation

SPF — sun protection factor

TGF — transforming growth factor

Th — T-helper cells

TRT — thermal relaxation time

TIMP — tissue inhibitors of metalloproteinases

TLR — Toll-like receptors

TNF — tumor necrosis factor

TRP — transient receptor potential channel

TRPV — transient receptor potential vanilloid receptor

TRPA — transient receptor potential ankyrin receptor

TSLP — thymic stromal lipoprotein

UV — ultraviolet

UVA — ultraviolet type A

UVB — ultraviolet type B

VEGF — vascular endothelial growth factor

VIP — vasoactive intestinal peptide

WGS — genome sequencing

WES — whole exome sequencing

Introduction

Rosacea and couperosis are two of the most common causes of red skin. Could this be a big problem? It can. For many people worldwide (on average, one in twenty people suffer from rosacea), it is a problem that significantly impacts their quality of life. It's hard to hide transient or persistent facial redness that gives away your excitement or gives the impression that you're worried. It worsens after going to a restaurant, a walk in the sun, or a visit to the bathhouse. People with rosacea are often mistaken for alcoholics, even if they are utterly intolerant of alcohol, and are thus treated with prejudice.

In 2018, Galderma conducted a large-scale study to assess how the presence of rosacea affects people's lives. This work focused not on the clinical symptoms but on the emotional, psychological, and social difficulties faced by people with this pathology.

Participants included 710 rosacea patients (34% men, 66% women, mean age 44.5 ± 13.8) and 554 physicians supervising people with rosacea from six countries (France, Germany, Italy, the UK, Canada, and the USA). The study findings were subsequently published in the *Rosacea: Beyond The Visible* report, and demonstrated the significant impact of rosacea on patients' quality of life. Another study aim was to understand how much effort these people spend to hide their condition and how little the public knows about it. Here are the most significant findings from this report:

- 87% of patients complained of the presence of flare-ups of redness
- 22% had no flare-ups, but reported high levels of discomfort due to other symptoms
- 59% reported persistent symptoms, with no periods of decline or remission, despite multiple visits to doctors and use of various medications over the years
- 22% noted the absence of outbreaks

- 14% did not report any manifestations of the disease at the time of the survey
- 1% said they had not noticed any rosacea manifestations in the last year
- In 46% of cases, symptoms were present almost constantly and worsened during outbreaks
- All patients frequently visited doctors, with 18% even calling for emergency services and 29% feeling that doctors did not take them seriously
- According to patients, physicians underestimated the importance of their complaints, such as (in decreasing order of underestimation) rough skin, pain, dryness, scaling, itching, burning, eye symptoms, edema, transient redness, burning, and redness of the nose
- At the same time, physicians overestimated the impact of the presence of papules and pustules, dilated vessels, persistent redness, and flare-ups on patients' quality of life
- In 37% of cases, patients complained that family and friends did not realize how severely they were impacted by rosacea, mainly because the patients themselves preferred to hide the problems for fear of judgment or misunderstanding
- A third of those surveyed have lost their self-confidence
- One in four felt annoyed
- One in ten was depressed
- One in five stated that they had to make significant changes in their lives to control rosacea
- In 86% of cases, restrictions were made to diet, sports, traveling to warm countries and generally being in the sun, using cosmetics, etc., which significantly affected their life comfort
- 82% of respondents believed that they were not in control of the disease, despite avoiding triggers of exacerbations and complying with treatment
- 55% stated that having rosacea affected their productivity at work
- 76% said having rosacea affected their quality of life
- Some people rated this impact as very pronounced (22%) or almost catastrophic (9%)

Although we do not have data to estimate the prevalence and impact of couperosis on quality of life, it is likely that all aforementioned complaints apply to this condition to a greater or lesser extent, since these two pathologies go side by side. In clinical practice, they are also often confused, which is why we will consider them together in this edition. This book will delve into the causes of these diseases and the range of potential treatments, aiming to significantly ease the life of patients with rosacea and couperosis.

Part I

Rosacea

Rosacea is a chronic, recurrent facial skin disease caused by angioneurotic disorders, which are polyetiological and are characterized by a staged course. To this definition, we could add "progressive, inflammatory, with no specific clinical features."

On average, rosacea is thought to affect about 5% of adults worldwide, with the estimates ranging from 1% to 20% (Tan J. et al., 2013). While rosacea was previously thought to be a disease of people of Celtic phototype, current evidence shows that rosacea occurs in people of all phototypes. However, in fair-skinned patients it is much more noticeable, due to which they are more likely to seek help in the early stages of the disease, while people with dark skin come to doctors already having signs of progression (Gallo R.L. et al., 2017).

Rosacea starts after the age of 30, with peak incidence in the 40s and 50s. As older people are becoming more numerous due to global population aging, the overall incidence is on the rise. Men tend to be more often and more severely affected than women, but women are more concerned about their appearance and more likely to seek medical help. The phymatous form of rosacea occurs almost exclusively in men (Gether L. et al., 2018).

Chapter 1
Etiology and pathogenesis

Rosacea is one of those diseases for which the exact mechanism has not yet been established. Indeed, many links are involved in the pathogenesis of rosacea, which are still being studied. It is currently believed that rosacea is caused by a combination of immune system disorders, changes in vascular reactivity, abnormalities in the perception and transmission of nerve signals, deterioration of skin barrier function, and microflora dysbiosis against the background of genetic predisposition, which ultimately leads to increased skin sensitivity, inflammation, and vascular dilation. It is important to note that this is the **combination of contributing factors**, and in many cases the processes are cross-reacting.

1.1. Immune factor

It is well established that rosacea patients have a **compromised innate immune system**. Innate immunity is the body's innate ability to respond to various external influences, mainly microorganisms. a key role in innate immunity is played by toll-like receptors (TLR; in the skin, it is TLR2) and the cathelicidin pathway (Kligman A.M., 2004).

TLR2 is a class of transmembrane cell receptors, the detecting part of which is located on the surface of epithelial cells (including keratinocytes) and immune system cells (monocytes/macrophages, neutrophils, dendritic and mast cells). When they encounter various structures of microorganisms, receptors are activated and immune response is triggered inside the cell. This initiates a chain reaction with the release of pro-inflammatory cytokines, chemokines, proteases, and pro-angiogenic factors aimed at fighting the foreign pathogen. The central link in this fight is the antimicrobial peptide cathelicidin (CAMP) and its active form peptide LL-37, the action of which is associated with increased inflammation in the skin, dilation of existing vessels, and activation of the synthesis of new ones (angiogenesis) through vascular endothelial growth factor (VEGF), increased neutrophil chemotaxis, as well as dysregulation of the synthesis of extracellular matrix components. TLR2 activation increases cathelicidin synthesis as well as trypsin-like serine protease kallikrein 5 (KLK5), the enzyme by which cathelicidin is converted to LL-37 (Tan J. et al., Berg M., 2013; Scheenstra M.R. et al., 2020).

In rosacea, TLR2 become particularly susceptible to microorganisms, resulting in abnormal release of pro-inflammatory cytokines and antimicrobial peptides. Compared with normal skin, skin affected by rosacea is characterized by significantly higher cathelicidin expression and thousands of times higher levels of proteases in the *stratum corneum* that activate cathelicidins. The LL-37 and KLK5 molecules also differ from those in normal skin, as TLR2 in rosacea patients begin to respond to microorganisms and many other triggering factors, such as heat/cold, ultraviolet (UV) radiation, and alcohol.

Other components of innate immunity, such as NOD-like receptor protein 3 (NLRP3) inflammasomes (a multiprotein complex that plays a pivotal role in regulating the innate immune system and inflammatory signaling) and protease-activated transmembrane receptor 2 (PAR2) responsible for activating the inflammatory response, are also involved (Segovia J. et al., 2012). PAR2 also mediates neuroinflammation, itch and pain, T-cell recruitment, mast cell degranulation, vasodilation, and the release of many pro-inflammatory agents (Steinhoff M. et al., 2005). The expression of both TLR2 and PAR2 is upregulated in the skin of rosacea patients (Yamasaki K. et al., 2011; Kim J.Y. et al., 2014).

As a result, abnormal amounts of LL-37 drive a range of responses (**Fig. I-1-1**) (Buddenkotte J. et al., 2018; Scheenstra M.R. et al., 2020):

- Formation of new vessels and impairment of vascular function in general due to VEGF activation and sphingosine-1-phosphate expression. The latter is a signaling sphingolipid which, in addition to stimulation of angiogenesis, also increases vascular permeability.
- Mast cell degranulation through interaction with transient receptor potential vanilloid 4 (TRPV4) receptors with subsequent vasodilation and maintenance of the inflammatory response.

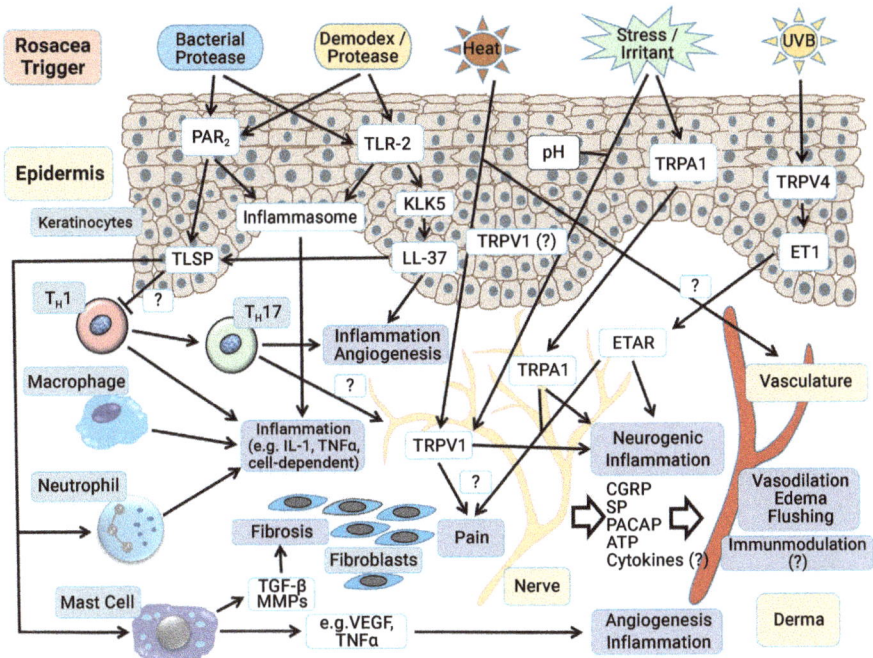

Figure I-1-1. Rosacea pathogenesis (adapted from Buddenkotte J. et al., 2018)

- Stimulation of a shift in the T-cell response to a predominance of type 17 T-helper cells through suppression of thymic stromal lipoprotein (TSLP).
- Neutrophil chemotaxis through the induction of interleukin (IL) 8. Neutrophils are the primary source of reactive oxygen species (ROS) with which they fight pathogens. Excessive ROS amounts hurt the skin through multiple processes — oxidative stress is one of the main pathogenetic links in rosacea.
- Triggering fibrosis processes directly through action on fibroblasts and indirectly through action on mast cells.

Separately, we would like to focus on some new aspects of immune reactions as they open up promising approaches in treating rosacea.

1.1.1. IL-17 and T-cell immunity imbalance

Recent studies indicate that IL-17, a pro-inflammatory cytokine produced by T-helper cells, has angiogenic activity and plays a significant role in the pathogenesis of rosacea. In perivascular skin infiltrates of patients with all forms of rosacea, many T-helper type 1 (Th1) and 17 (Th17) cells, as well as macrophages and mast cells in the areas of papules and erythema, and neutrophils in pustules were found. T-cell activity and IL-17 immunostaining were significantly higher in the skin of rosacea patients compared to the skin of lupus patients and healthy individuals, with the greatest prevalence of the papulopustular form, followed by phymatous and erythematotelangiectatic forms (Buhl T. et al., 2015).

Increased gene expression of IL-6, tumor necrosis factor (TNF), IL-20, and CCL2, all of which stimulate IL-17 and IL-22 synthesis, was also detected. IL-6 deserves special attention because it not only directly stimulates IL-17 release but also participates in a positive feedback loop and enhances Th17 differentiation, leading to a further increase in IL-17 (Buhl T. et al., 2015).

It was previously assumed that only T-cells could produce IL-17. Still, there is now evidence that other cells of the immune system — macrophages, dendritic cells, natural killer cells, and neutrophils — are also capable of producing it. Neutrophils are thought to make an important contribution to the development of inflammation in rosacea, and the formation of pustules is a clinical manifestation of their penetration into the perifollicular space (Speeckaert R. et al., 2016).

The shift towards predominance of Th1/Th17 cells in inflammatory infiltrates of rosacea patients may be associated with *Demodex* mites. The fact is that *Bacillus oleronius* bacteria, which are found in *D. folliculorum mites*, act as chemotactic agents for neutrophils and can stimulate the release of IL-17 by neutrophils. In addition, when skin samples from patients with increased *D. folliculorum* densities were analyzed, increased levels of cytokines such as IL-8, IL-1β and TNFα were found. IL-1β has been shown to play a key role in the differentiation of Th17 (Lasigliè D. et al., 2011; Speeckaert R. et al., 2016).

1.1.2. Mast cells

Mast cells are another representative of the immune system cells. They are present in various tissues, and their number is particularly high in mucous membranes and skin, where they comprise 10% of all immunocompetent cells.

Mast cells are among the first to interact with environmental antigens and allergens as well as invasive pathogens. Once activated, mast cells promote the release of various mediators and significantly impact the pathophysiology of inflammatory diseases. One such mediator is histamine, a compound that accounts for the increase in vascular wall permeability, influx of inflammatory elements, and the appearance of pruritus (Varricchi G. et al., 2019).

Recent studies have shown that the number of mast cells in patients with papulopustular and erythematous-telangiectatic forms of rosacea is significantly higher than in those with unaffected skin. a positive correlation was also observed between mast cell density and rosacea duration (Ahn C.S., Huang W.W., 2018).

The mechanisms of interaction between mast cells and other immune cells — including macrophages, neutrophils, and T-cells — in rosacea, are poorly understood. However, it has been shown that other immune cells can activate mast cells or activate neighboring cells by releasing pro-inflammatory mediators. It is also known that brimonidine and botulinum toxin, which are used in rosacea therapy, reduce mast cell migration and inhibit mast cell degranulation, resulting in reduced inflammation and symptom relief (Kim M. et al., 2017; Wang L. et al., 2020). Preclinical studies conducted by Dr. Richard Gallo and colleagues at the University of California also support the role of mast cells. In their cohorts, using a mast cell stabilizer effectively reduced the development of rosacea-like inflammation (Gallo R.L. et al., 2018).

In addition to histamine, mast cells release many other active substances, including IL-1, -4, -13, transforming growth factor (TGF)β, TNFα, VEGF, proteases, and others. In addition to inflammatory reactions, they are also involved in cell proliferation, angiogenesis, and regulation of extracellular matrix homeostasis.

According to recent data, mast cells participate in the development of fibrosis in different organs (Brown M., O'Reilly S., 2019) and are actively involved in collagen synthesis (Atiakshin D. et al., 2020). Thus, some mediators released by mast cells directly stimulate fibroblasts' synthetic function and migration. Mast cells synthesize glycosaminoglycans, which change the microenvironment of fibroblasts and indirectly influence their activity (Atiakshin D. et al., 2020). Proteases secreted by mast cells can modify the ratio of matrix metalloproteinases (MMP) and their tissue inhibitors (TIMP), which also affects the fibrinolysis and fibrino-genesis processes. The morphology of collagen fibrils that are formed as a result depends on the pH of the medium, whereby an increase in pH to 7.6–8.1 leads to an enlargement of the fibril diameter by almost one order of magnitude. This observation is of practical value in developing the therapeutic approaches to wound management.

Based on all the above, it can be concluded that mast cells play a role in the development of erythematous inflammatory symptoms of rosacea but also contribute to tissue overgrowth, i.e., progression to phymatous forms.

1.1.3. Neurovascular dysfunction and neurogenic inflammation

The reaction to typical stimuli in patients with rosacea is more pro-nounced than in healthy people and has peculiarities. In the initial stages, it manifests as transient redness, which eventually becomes persistent. Erythema is associated with vascular dysfunction, manifest-ed as vasodilation (vasodilation). Only after some time, inflammation accompanies the erythema due to impaired skin immunity. To empha-size the causal relationship, this type of inflammation is denoted as **neurogenic** (Sulk M. et al., 2012; Kucher A.N., 2020).

There is increasing evidence that neurogenic inflammation may be the key to unlocking the secret of rosacea and one of the main thera-peutic targets. However, it is worth noting that neurogenic inflamma-tion is present in the pathogenesis of some other chronic inflamma-tory diseases and pathological conditions of the skin, such as psoriasis, atopic dermatitis, skin, and hypertrophic scars (Rosa A.C., Fantozzi R, 2013; Marek-Jozefowicz L. et al., 2023).

Sensory receptors of cells

Neurogenic inflammation in the skin begins with a massive release of neurotransmitters from nerve endings in response to noninfec-tious stimuli such as solar radiation, alcohol, spicy food, hot drinks, heat/cold, cosmetics, psychoemotional stress, etc. The perception of these stimuli by cells is the responsibility of special sensory receptors on cell membranes (Yamasaki K. et al., 2009; Del Rosso J.Q., 2012).

Special sensory receptors on cell membranes are responsible for cells' perception of these stimuli (Yamasaki K. et al., 2009; Del Rosso J.Q., 2012). These include cation channels with transient receptor potential (TRP channels), in particular, vanilloid receptors (TRPV) and ankyrin receptor type 1 (TRPA1).

These receptors are found on many cells in the skin, including sensitive neurons, keratinocytes, fibroblasts, blood vessels, immunocytes, mast cells, and other tissues, including the intestine cells.

Four subtypes of TRPV receptors have been described. TRPV1 regulates vascular tone and pain perception, activated by capsaicin, heat, and inflammation. TRPV2 plays a role in innate immunity, regulation of vascular tone, pain perception, inflammation, and thermal sensitivity. TRPV3 and TRPV4 are responsible for thermal sensitivity (Ni Raghallaigh S., Powell F.C., 2014). The erythematous form of rosacea is characterized by increased expression of TRPV1, TRPV2, and TRPV3 genes. While rosacea papulopustulosa is associated with an increased immunoreactivity of TRPV2 and TRPV4, in rhinophyma such immunoreactivity is observed in TRPV3 and TRPV4 (Sulk M. et al., 2012).

TRPA1 is activated by spices such as cinnamaldehyde, mustard oil, and thermal stimuli. In experiments on mice, topical cinnamaldehyde caused vasodilation via a TRPA1-dependent mechanism, which may be associated with the symptom of hyperemia in rosacea patients (Pozsgai G. et al., 2010). TRPA1 is also capable of responding to increased ROS levels, which may support the role of oxidative stress in the development of rosacea (Graepel R. et al., 2011). In rat neurons, TRPA1 colocalizes with PAR2, which can be activated by proteases and induce inflammation in human skin. Presumably, the increased amount of serine proteases in rosacea can induce TRPA1-mediated inflammation through the regulation of PAR (Dai Y. et al., 2007).

Other cellular receptors have also been shown to be involved in the rosacea pathogenesis, in particular TLR2 and PAR2 receptors of sensitive neurons (Buddenkotte J. et al., 2018; Storozhuk M.V., Zholos A.V., 2018).

Thus, the dysfunction of the cell receptor apparatus in rosacea makes the skin much more susceptible to a variety of external factors (Rainer B.M. et al., 2017). Hence, it is unsurprising that patients note increased skin sensitivity to heat/cold, cosmetics, and warm and cold water (Guzman-Sanchez D.A. et al., 2007).

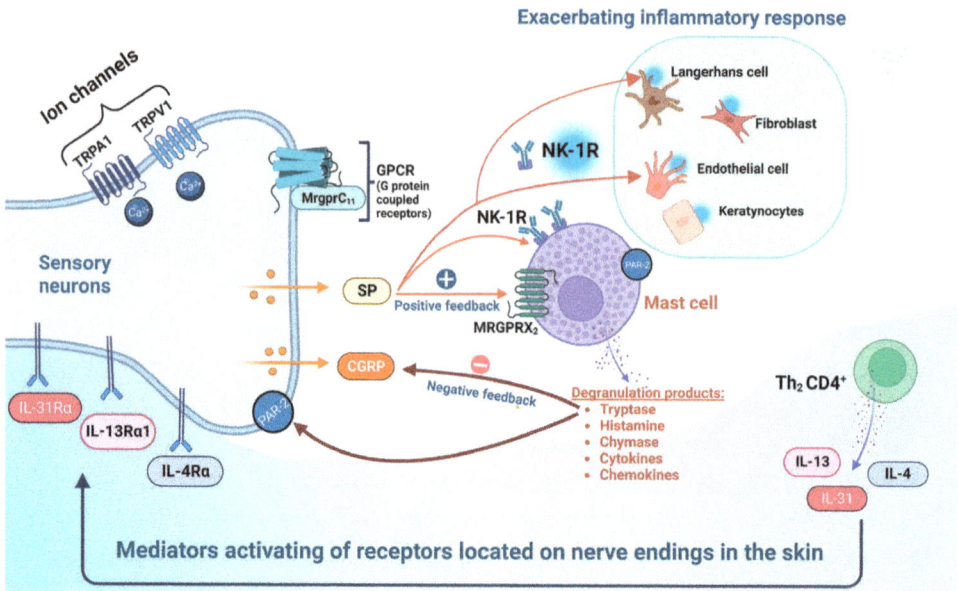

Figure I-1-2. Development of neurogenic inflammation in the skin (adapted from Marek-Jozefowicz L. et al., 2023)

Neurotransmitters

In response to external stimulation, skin cells release various biologically active substances mediated by diverse physiological processes (**Fig. I-1-2**) (Marek-Jozefowicz L. et al., 2023). Substances that are secreted by nerve endings are called neurotransmitters.

Some neurotransmitters such as substance P, pituitary adenylate cyclase-activating polypeptide (PACAP), vasoactive intestinal peptide (VIP), and calcitonin gene-related peptide (CGRP) directly relax smooth muscle cells of the vascular wall, dilating vessels, and promoting edema (Aubdool A.A., Brain S.D., 2011; Baylie R.L., Brayden J.E., 2011; Buddenkotte J., Steinhoff M., 2018). In addition, PACAP can stimulate NO release from endothelial cells, resulting in indirect vasodilation (Seeliger S. et al., 2010).

Neurotransmitters activate mast cells, which in response release histamine, causing vasodilation, and tryptase (a chemotactic agent for fibroblasts) contributing to the development of fibrosis in rosacea

(Muto Y. et al., 2014). Neurotransmitters stimulate IL-1β production and activate leukocyte migration by increasing the amount of vascular endothelial adhesion molecules in rosacea (Shi X. et al., 2011).

Genetic predisposition

The biologically active substances and receptors involved in the development of neurogenic inflammation are under genetic control.

Deng Z. et al. (2023) published the results of whole genome sequencing (WGS) performed in three large families of rosacea patients, along with the whole exome sequencing (WES) results pertaining to 49 families. Single rare variants in *LRRC4*, *SH3PXD2A*, and *SLC26A8* genes were identified in large families, while gene ontology analysis demonstrated that they encode proteins involved in neurosynaptic processes and cell adhesion (Deng Z. et al., 2023).

According to *in vitro* studies, mutations in *LRRC4*, *SH3PXD2A*, and *SLC26A8* trigger the production of vasoactive neuropeptides in human neurons. In a mouse model replicating a recurrent *LRRC4* mutation characteristic of rosacea patients, the authors observed rosacea-like skin inflammation based on excessive VIP release by peripheral neurons. These results confirm the presence of hereditary predisposition and a significant contribution of neurogenic inflammation to the development of rosacea, which considerably deepens the understanding of the etiopathogenesis of rosacea and contributes to the search for effective therapeutic approaches (**Fig. I-1-3**).

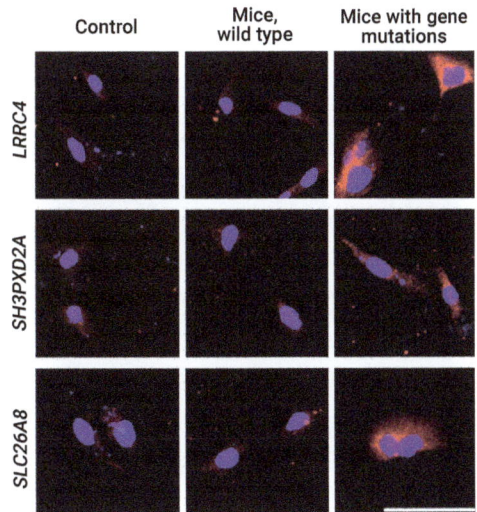

Figure I-1-3. *LRRC4/SH3PXD2A/SLC26A8* gene mutations increase the level of vasoactive neuropeptides released by nerve cells (adapted from Deng Z. et al., 2023)

1.2. Skin barrier function

Inflammation observed in rosacea is mainly attributed to the failure of *stratum corneum* to fulfill its protective function, due to which foreign agents begin to pass through it. Cells instantly react by defending the body with the help of inflammation.

Studies show that rosacea patients have a significantly increased rate of transepidermal water loss, a landmark parameter indicative of impaired skin barrier function. It is assumed that this process is associated with changes in the composition of sebum lipids, compromising the physiological balance of various fatty acids and causing increased permeability of the lipid barrier (Ní Raghallaigh S. et al., 2012). Thus, sebum of rosacea patients contains an increased concentration of myristic acid (C14:0) and lower levels of long-chain fatty acids — arachic acid (C20:0), behenic acid (C22:0), tricosanoic acid (C23:0), and lignoceric acid (C24:0) — compared to the composition of sebum in healthy people. In particular, myristic acid has a pronounced ability to increase the permeability of the skin barrier.

The imbalance of fatty acids in the composition of sebum is the leading cause of impaired skin barrier function in rosacea. This observation is confirmed by very low rosacea occurrence before puberty when the sebaceous glands are still underdeveloped, as well as by the therapeutic efficacy of low-dose isotretinoin, which reduces sebum and cyclic adenosine monophosphate (cAMP) production. In addition, altering the balance of fatty acids (in terms of nutrient environment and pH) can also promote the survival of pathogenic or opportunistic microorganisms on the skin and further enhance the production of antimicrobial peptides.

1.3. Microbiome

Microorganisms that live on the skin as well as those in the intestine are also implicated in the pathogenesis of rosacea.

1.3.1. Skin microbiome

For a long time, the mite *Demodex folliculorum*, which lives in the sebaceous glands, was claimed to be the leading cause of rosacea.

However, these perceptions have changed due to the greater recognition of the importance of the skin microbiome. While it is true that rosacea patients have a higher population of *D. folliculorum*, it is now established that they also have an imbalance in the microbial composition of the skin. Yet, it is still unclear whether this imbalance or the aforementioned phenomena is primary mechanism leading to the emergence of rosacea.

It has been suggested that components of the mite cell membrane activate TLR2, which increases KLK5 expression (Ferrer L. et al., 2014). But *D. folliculorum* is not the only pathogen, as in one study, skin colonization by this mite was reduced through the application of topical antibiotics without improvements in the rosacea symptoms (Koijak M. et al., 2002).

Since antibiotics are used to treat rosacea with a certain degree of success, the researchers suggested that bacteria may cause the disease. It has also been established that *Bacillus oleronius* — a fixed gram-negative microorganism isolated from *Demodex* mites — provokes the synthesis of allergenic proteins in patients with certain subtypes of rosacea (O'Reilly N. et al., 2012). In several studies, the production of matrix metalloproteinase-9 (MMP-9), TNFα, and IL-8 was increased in neutrophils "trained" by *Bacillus oleronius* antigens, which caused a sustained inflammatory response even in people without rosacea (Yamasaki K. et al., 2009; Two A.M. et al., 2015).

Studies exploring the role of the commensal *Staphylococcus epidermidis* further indicate that, in normal skin, it produces antimicrobial peptides that help humans prevent disease caused by pathogenic bacteria. But when placed on the skin with rosacea, *Staphylococcus epidermidis* synthesizes specific pathogenicity factors, leading to the activation of TLR2 and triggering the "cathelicidin–KLK5" inflammatory cascade (Ferrer L. et al., 2014).

Thus, it is currently believed that, since the innate immune system of rosacea patients is unable to properly recognize the "good" commensal microorganisms that live and multiply naturally on the skin (*Cutibacterium acnes*, *Staph. epidermidis*, *D. folliculorum*, etc.), it reacts to them as "enemies" by developing an inflammatory reaction. The resulting problems and changes in the composition of the skin microbiome of rosacea patients compared to the microbiome of healthy people may be due to the alterations in the sebum composition. Indeed, several authors have noted that, in rosacea, the number of bacteria of the genera *Corynebacterium*, *Actinomyces*, and *Cutibacterium* (known "lovers" of sebum) decreases significantly, and the number of *Actinobacteria* and *Firmicutis* types increases (Marson J.W. et al., 2020; Wang R. et al., 2020).

Another important finding in this context is that **the more the microbiome composition changes** (deviates from a balanced state), **the more the skin barrier function deteriorates** in the areas affected by rosacea (Yuan C. et al., 2020).

As with other factors implicated in the rosacea pathogenesis, a change in one parameter aggravates another and reactions take on a cyclical character.

1.3.2. Gut microbiome

In their 2017 study involving 50,000 patients, Egeberg A. and colleagues found that the prevalence of celiac disease, Crohn's disease, ulcerative colitis, *Helicobacter pilori* infection, bacterial overgrowth syndrome, and irritable bowel syndrome was higher in rosacea patients compared to controls. This association has been evaluated by other researchers but with conflicting results, given that a higher frequency of *H. pilori* infection in rosacea patients was reported by several authors (Diaz C. et al., 2003; Gravina A. et al., 2015).

H. pilori are gram-negative bacteria that can cause the development of chronic gastritis, gastric and duodenal ulcers, and gastric adenocarcinoma. In numerous studies, improvements in rosacea symptoms were observed after *Helicobacter* eradication. However, it is difficult to establish a pathogenetic link, as antibiotics are effective in treating any infectious disease.

In the study conducted by Egeberg A. et al. (2017), rosacea patients were 13 times more likely to have **bacterial overgrowth syndrome** than controls. Thus, the authors suggested that circulating cytokines, especially TNFα, played a role in the high prevalence of rosacea. Treatment of bacterial overgrowth syndrome with antibiotics in 40 patients that took part in the study conducted by Drago F. et al. (2016) resulted in remission of rosacea. Most participants maintained remission for three years.

In general, the gastrointestinal microbiome is an exciting target for rosacea treatment. However, this approach has several problems, including the considerable variability in the microbial community among individuals. Factors influencing these differences include genetics, diet, environmental conditions, and hygiene habits, among others. Accordingly, further research on a global scale is needed in this domain (Gupta V.K. et al., 2017).

Another interesting issue in this context is the association between **inflammatory bowel disease** and rosacea. In their nationwide study conducted in Taiwan, which involved more than 89,000 patients with rosacea, such association was determined (Wu C.-Y. et al., 2017). These findings correlated with data obtained in Danish and American studies (Li W.Q. et al., 2016).

1.4. Genetic predisposition

The higher incidence of rosacea in fair-skinned people of European descent indicates that specific genes are associated with this condition. However, until recently, these genes were not known. Exciting data was obtained owing to 23andme, a genetic testing company. Analysis of their database has revealed specific gene variants associated with rosacea — these are the genes encoding butyrophilin-like protein 2 and human leukocyte antigen DRA. Both genes are associated with the adaptive immune system, confirming the central role of immune dysregulation in the pathogenesis of rosacea (Chang A.L.S. et al., 2015).

Another study has shown the role of the glutathione-S-transferase gene, one of the central enzymes of the antioxidant system. The authors found that, as this gene is defective in rosacea patients, their antioxidant defense system is not as effective as in healthy people (Woo Y.R. et al., 2016). In addition to the fact that other links in the pathogenesis of rosacea are associated with excessive amounts of ROS in the skin, oxidative stress is posited to be a very significant player in the emergence and progression of the disease.

There is a long-standing theory that all pathogenetic links of rosacea converge into the so-called stress of the endoplasmic reticulum (Plewig G., Kilgman A.M., 2019). As this organelle is responsible for synthesizing and transporting proteins, lipids, and steroids, its problems adversely affect the whole cell and the body. Some scholars believe that the stress of the endoplasmic reticulum underlies all further "breakdowns" in rosacea. However, this theory is not widely supported by scientific evidence.

1.5. Rosacea-contributing factors

1.5.1. Triggering factors

Despite the insufficiently understood pathogenesis of rosacea, doctors and patients "with experience" know that this disease has many provoking factors (triggers), including high temperature, sun exposure, spicy food, alcohol consumption, physical exertion, and feelings of anger or embarrassment. Some triggers, such as high temperature, directly affect the blood vessels by vasodilating them. Others, as we have discussed, utilize different mechanisms that ultimately lead to the development of inflammation in the skin.

Insolation is one of the most cited triggers for facial hot flashes and worsening of rosacea symptoms (**Fig. I-1-4**). In this case, exacerbations are thought to result from the following processes:
1. The abovementioned action of ultraviolet (UV) radiation on TRPV receptors with subsequent triggering of neurogenic inflammation.
2. Vitamin D causes increased expression of cathelicidin in keratinocytes, which triggers a cascade of inflammatory responses.
3. UVB rays stimulate skin vascular proliferation through the induction of fibroblast growth factor 2 (FGF-2) and VEGF-2 (Bielenberg D.R. et al., 1998).
4. After excessive UV exposure, more ROS are generated in the skin, further supporting the KLK5–cathelicidin inflammatory cascade (Yamasaki K. et al., 2009).
5. Matrix metalloproteinases MMP-1, -3 and -9, which increase in quantity under UV exposure, damage the intercellular substance of the dermis and blood vessels.

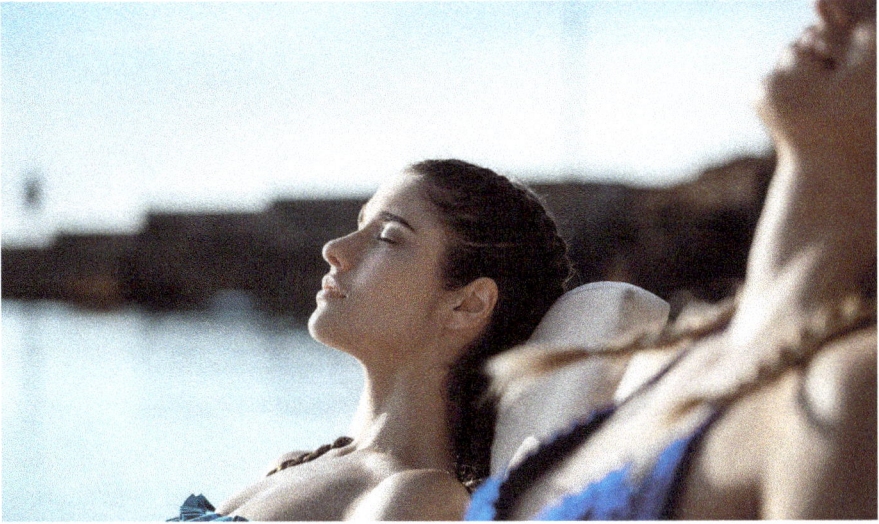

Figure I-1-4. Sun exposure can aggravate rosacea
(Image by cooki_studio, Freepik.com)

Avoiding prolonged sun exposure and using proper protection (not only cosmetics, but also clothing and head cover) can help these patients prevent rosacea exacerbations. Interestingly, despite the sensitivity to the sun, rosacea patients are less likely to have pigmentary disorders than the average population, but the reason for this distinction is still unclear.

In addition to insolation, intolerance of certain **foods** is often mentioned by patients. In the survey conducted by the National Rosacea Society of the United States (the US National Rosacea Society), 78% of more than 400 patients changed their diet because of the disease. In addition, 95% of this group subsequently experienced reduced exacerbations (Harper J., 2005).

The main provoking factors associated with food intake are:
- Extreme (hot or high) temperature
- Alcohol
- Capsaicin
- Cinnamaldehyde

3% of rosacea patients described hot coffee as a trigger for exacerbation, and 30% mentioned hot tea. Wine consumption triggered exacerbations in 52% of patients and hard alcohol in 42%. The most frequently mentioned triggers included spices (75%), hot sauces (54%), and hot (47%) and red peppers (37%), all of which contain capsaicin (**Fig. I-1-5**). As cinnamaldehyde is found in cinnamon, chocolate, and some seemingly unrelated foods (tomatoes, citrus fruits), these are often poorly tolerated by rosacea patients. Indeed, in the survey conducted by Scheman A. et al. (2013), tomatoes were blamed for exacerbating rosacea symptoms by 30% of respondents, chocolate by 23%, and citrus fruits by 22%.

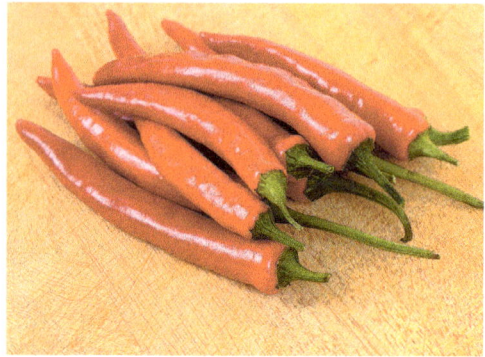

Figure I-1-5. Capsaicin from hot pepper negatively affects rosacea (Image by kstudio, Freepik.com)

It should be noted that recent studies counter the previous view that coffee exacerbates rosacea symptoms. The basis for this change in perspective was the analysis of data from one of the most extensive epidemiological studies — Nurses' Health Study II (NHS II), monitoring the health of more than a 100,000 female nurses for decades. During their work, Li S. et al. (2018) studied the health status of 82,737 NHS II participants, among whom 4,945 had rosacea.

After analyzing various risk factors (and adjusting for them), the authors came to an unexpected conclusion. Among those women who drank four or more cups of coffee a day, the probability of developing rosacea was 23% lower compared to those who indulged in a cup of this drink less than once a month. No such association was found for decaffeinated coffee (Li S. et al., 2018).

Recently, many scientists started talking about the positive effects of caffeine on various aspects of human health. For example, caffeine constricts blood vessels in the skin and has an anti-inflammatory effect, potentially reducing the risk of rosacea. However, as this beverage is usually consumed hot, it can cause erythema flare-ups.

Other common triggering factors of rosacea are stress, local irritants, medications (vasodilators, nicotinic acid), and endocrine, nervous, and gastrointestinal diseases. Smoking also has a negative impact on symptom manifestation (Wang Y. et al., 2020).

In a survey conducted by the US National Rosacea Society, 1,066 patients were asked to note the 10 most frequent triggers that cause their disease to worsen, and the findings are shown in **Table I-1-1**.

Table I-1-1. Prevalence of rosacea triggers (Harper J., 2005)

FACTORS	PARTICIPANTS, %
Sun exposure	81
Emotional stress	79
Hot weather	75
Wind	57
Heavy exercise	56
Alcohol consumption	52
Hot baths	51
Cold weather	46
Spicy food	45
Humidity	44

1.5.2. Risk factors and comorbidities

The pathogenesis of rosacea involves many pathologic mechanisms, some of which are systemic. The same disorders are involved in the pathogenesis of other diseases. Recent studies have shown that patients with rosacea are more likely than healthy people to have diseases of the digestive, nervous, cardiovascular and immune systems, as well as mental health problems.

Links between rosacea and the following pathologies (Haber R., El Gemayel M., 2018) have now been confirmed:
- Type 1 diabetes (predominantly in women)
- Crohn's disease
- Ulcerative colitis
- Celiac disease
- Multiple sclerosis

- Migraine
- Parkinson's disease
- Alzheimer's disease
- Dementia
- Thyroid cancer
- Squamous cell carcinoma
- Glioma
- Rheumatoid arthritis

Rosacea patients have a significantly increased risk of developing depression, but whether the mechanism here is pathogenetic or psychological is not fully understood (Heisig M., Reich A., 2018).

In addition to comorbidities, several disorders that increase the risk of rosacea have been identified. Thus, according to the Korean national database of medical examinations, which includes information on almost 3,000,000 people, the likelihood of rosacea (at least in Korean population) was increased if they had the following metabolic disorders (Kim J. et al., 2019):

- Arterial hypertension (BP >130/85 mmHg) — 1.2 times
- Hyperglycemia — 1.38 times
- Hypertriglyceridemia — 1.06 times
- Low content of high-density lipoproteins — 1.51 times
- Increase in waist circumference (> 90 cm in men and > 85 cm in women) — 1.33 times

Chapter 2
Classification and clinical manifestation

2.1. Classification

As there is currently no generally accepted classification of rosacea, one of the two main variants is typically adopted in research and practice.

In 2002, the US National Rosacea Society assembled an expert committee to develop the first standard classification of rosacea. This classification allocates four disease phenotypes according to **clinical symptoms** (Wilkin J. et al., 2002):

- Erythematotelangiectatic (centrofacial)
- Papulopustular (inflammatory, acne-like)
- Glandular hyperplastic (phymas)
- Ocular (ophthalmorosacea)

There is also a classification based on **the course of the disease**. Accordingly, the following stages are distinguished:

- **Pre-rosacea (disease onset):** Periodic facial redness due to various triggering factors, which may exist for several years before progressing to the next stage.
- **Erythematous stage:** Persistent facial erythema with flashes of redness under the influence of triggering factors. There may be a sensation of warmth, and localization is limited to the central part of the face and nasolabial folds.
- **Papular stage:** Bright erythema, thickened skin in the affected area, telangiectasia, and inflammatory rashes (papules, nodules). Isolated or grouped pink rashes 3–5 mm in diameter, dense, with rounded outlines and blurred borders. Nodules are noticeable

due to more intense coloration. a smooth, sometimes shiny surface characterizes papules which are often covered with delicate scales. Infiltration is noted at the base of the most significant elements. Localization of papules on the cheeks, forehead, and chin, and sometimes in the area above the upper lip. Their number varies from single to multiple. The papules exist for many days or weeks and are not inclined to merge. Sometimes, papules are formed on an unchanged background. Patients are bothered by itching, fever, or burning in the facial area. Often, itching is not as pronounced in the areas of rashes but on their periphery — in the upper part of the forehead, cheekbones, lateral cheeks, and on the anterior surface of the neck. This phenomenon is particularly pronounced during the period of rash regression.

- **Pustular stage:** With further disease progression, many nodules undergo suppuration, forming papules 1–5 mm in size with yellow or greenish-yellow content. Pustules are formed in the erythema zone, but their appearance outside its boundaries is possible. Elements tend to cluster, especially in the nose, nasolabial folds, and chin. Over time, the lesion spreads from the central area to the skin of the forehead (up to the hairline) and cheeks. With this localization, papulopustular elements are often accompanied by significant itching. In the acute course of the disease, there is marked facial swelling, which is especially noticeable in the eyelid area, due to which the eye slits are narrowed.

- **Infiltrative productive stage (phyma):** Inflammatory nodules, infiltrate, tumor-like growths, and abundance of persistently dilated vessels emerge. Tumor-like growths are formed due to the progressive hyperplasia of sebaceous glands and connective tissue. These changes primarily affect the nose and the cheeks, creating a pronounced disfiguring effect.

This classification has helped systematize rosacea symptoms and has significantly improved patient care. However, it has some notable shortcomings, such as its failure to account for other symptoms of rosacea not described by clinical forms as well as for the "overlap" among subtypes.

Specific forms of rosacea have also been identified (Wilkin J. et al., 2002):

- Rosacea granulomatosa
- Steroid dermatitis
- Rosacea gram-negative
- Rosacea conglobata
- Rosacea fulminants

The critical insights into the pathogenesis of rosacea that have emerged over the past ten years have changed the understanding of the disease. Consequently, in 2017, the US National Rosacea Society Expert Committee proposed an updated classification that emphasized a more patient-centered **phenotypic** approach (Gallo R.L. et al., 2018).

According to this approach, **at least one diagnostic feature or two primary features are sufficient to diagnose** rosacea (**Table I-2-1**). Therefore, secondary signs in any number are not the criteria for diagnosis but may complement the diagnostic and primary signs. The specific type, approach to therapy, and the severity of the disease will depend on the combination of signs from all three major groups. Although many specialists still work according to the old classification, the transition from the division of rosacea into subtypes to phenotypes will allow the selection of more individualized treatments according to the characteristic features, rather than categorization by predetermined forms.

Table I-2-1. Symptoms, which are the basis of the 2017 classification of rosacea by the US National Rosacea Society (Gallo R.L. et al., 2018)

DIAGNOSTIC FEATURES	PRIMARY FEATURES	SECONDARY FEATURES
• Persistent centro-facial erythema aggravated by triggering factors • Phymatous changes	• Hot flashes/transient erythema • Inflammatory papules and pustules • Telangiectasias • Ocular manifestations: — Telangiectasias along the eyelid margin — Conjunctival injection (redness and dilation of blood vessels at the vaults of the conjunctiva, i.e., around the perimeter of the eyeball) — Blepharitis, keratitis, conjunctivitis, and sclerokeratitis	• Burning • Tingling sensation • Edema • Skin dryness

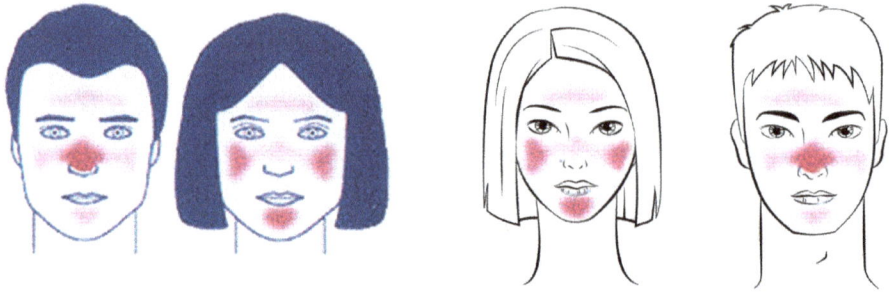

Figure I-2-1. Typical rosacea-affected areas in women and men

2.2. Clinical picture

2.2.1. General characterization

Rosacea is a facial skin pathology that:
- has a chronic, recurring course
- is due to angioedema
- is progressive and staggered
- has rashes localized over inactive muscles, so muscle contraction does not drain the resulting edema (the skin in these areas does not gather into folds due to edema)

Localization of the affected areas differs between women and men. In women, the cheeks and chin are mainly affected, while in men, the nose is the most affected part of the face (**Fig. I-2-1**).

It is important to emphasize that rosacea does not resolve spontaneously, but rather progresses through its successive stages (**Fig. I-2-2**). However, the rate of progression and the severity of clinical signs are individualized.

2.2.2. Clinical manifestation of rosacea according to the 2002 classification

Since most specialists are still working according to the 2002 classification of rosacea, in this section we will first present the clinical forms according to this classification and then describe the clinical features proposed in the 2017 classification.

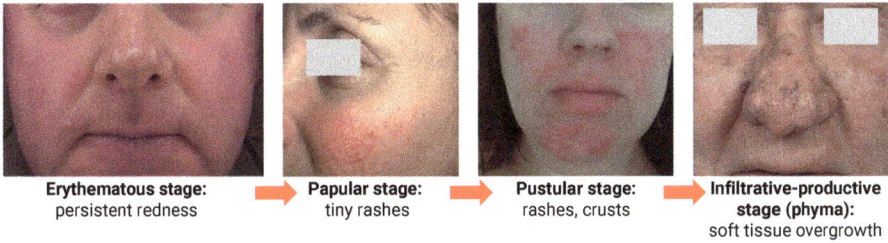

Erythematous stage: persistent redness ➡ Papular stage: tiny rashes ➡ Pustular stage: rashes, crusts ➡ Infiltrative-productive stage (phyma): soft tissue overgrowth

Figure I-2-2. Rosacea progression

According to the 2002 classification, persistent erythema in the central part of the face that has existed for three months is considered a mandatory clinical sign of rosacea.

Optional attributes include:

- Telangiectasias
- Papules
- Pustules
- Phymatous changes

Thus, the **only criterion for the diagnosis of rosacea, according to the 2002 classification, is persistent erythema of the central part of the face that has persisted for at least three months**. The other signs are also considered to establish the stages/forms of the disease.

Pre-rosacea

In this stage, the intermittent midface redness as a result of triggers is the primary symptom.

A legitimate question thus arises: *Are all those who blush easily from shame, heat, or alcohol intake candidates for rosacea diagnosis or not? Is it necessary to initiate treatment at this stage so that pre-rosacea does not turn into rosacea?*

Albert Kligman believed that not all redness should be considered pre-rosacea, as the diagnosis depends on the timing and extent of the erythema. If the redness lasts for more than five minutes, it is probably pre-rosacea. If the erythema spreads to the neck and upper chest, it is not pre-rosacea (recall that rosacea affects only the middle part of the face) (Kligman A.M., 2004).

Erythematotelangiectatic rosacea

This form is characterized by persistent stagnant erythema of varying intensity in the middle part of the face (**Fig. I-2-3**). Under the influence of triggering factors, the face suddenly becomes even redder (erythema flare), slowly returning to its original state. Often, noticeable changes in complexion occur several times during the appointment when the patient is agitated.

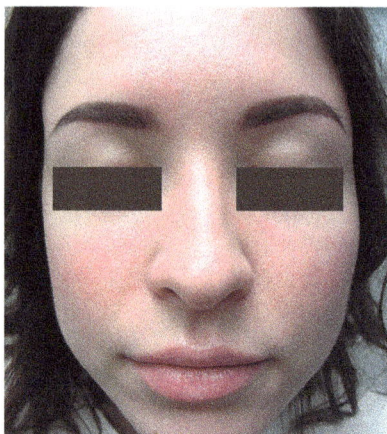

Figure I-2-3. Patient N., 32 years old. Erythema of the middle part of the face, multiple telangiectasias (Photo: Albanova V.I.)

Within the reddened skin are dilated small vessels (telangiectasias) supporting the redness, so erythema is called vascular. Subjective signs are burning and tingling. Erythema is often accompanied by swelling that appears or worsens during an outbreak. Skin roughness and slight desquamation may be present (**Table I-2-2**).

It is important to note that **erythema is caused by dysregulation of blood vessels, i.e., disruption of their function, while telangiectasias are structural changes in blood vessels**. This is why erythema

Table I-2-2. Severity of the erythematotelangiectatic rosacea

SYMPTOM	MILD	MODERATE	SEVERE
Erythema	Not persistent at first, but gradually become persistent	Moderately persistent	Expressed
Flushes (episodes of sudden redness)	Rare	Frequent	Frequent, prolonged
Telangiectasias	Small, barely noticeable	Notable	Multiple, prominent

can be treated with vasoconstrictors while telangiectasias cannot.

Papulopustular (inflammatory) rosacea

Isolated or grouped hemispherical pink papules surrounded by erythema coronae and pustules with yellowish contents first appear in the middle part of the face, then on the chin, forehead area up to and even crossing the hairline, behind the ears, and on the neck (**Fig. I-2-4**).

The presence of inflammatory papules and pustules aggravates the erythema. The papules and pustules may be painful and persistent (lasting for days to weeks), with residual redness but no scarring. The skin thickens, and large nodules and infiltrates appear (**Fig. I-2-5**). Telangiectasias may not be visible against erythema, papules, and pustules (**Table I-2-3**).

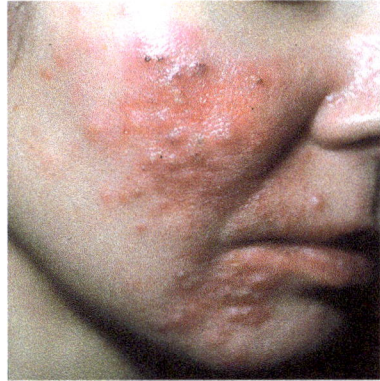

Figure I-2-4. Patient N., 35 years old. Grouped pink papules and pustules with yellowish content on the background of congestive hyperemia (Photo: Albanova V.I.)

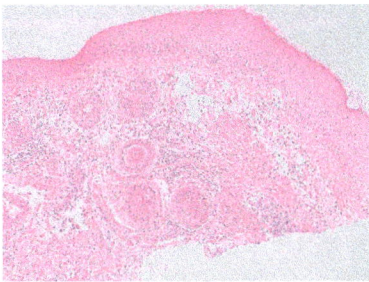

Figure I-2-5. Histology of the skin affected by rosacea papulopustulosa (adapted from Celiker H. et al., 2017)

A skin biopsy showed rosacea as enlarged, dilated capillaries and venules in the upper dermis, telangiectasias, perivascular and perifollicular lymphocytic infiltration, and superficial dermal edema. Concurrently, there is also solar elastosis (H&E; 100×)

Table I-2-3. Severity of the rosacea papulopustulosa

MILD	MODERATE	SEVERE
Small number of papules/pustules	Moderate number of papules/pustules	Multiple papules/pustules, may coalesce into plaques

Phymatous rosacea

In male patients, due to the hyperplasia of connective tissue, the skin becomes porous, thickened, increases in volume, and nodular growths appear, distorting the contours of the nose or other parts of the face. Such growths are called phymas.

Depending on the localization, phymas have different names, but rhinophyma (nose) is the most common (**Fig. I-2-6**). Less common are:

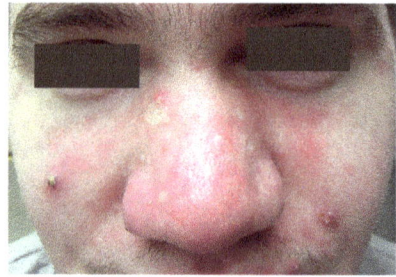

Figure I-2-6. Nodular formations in the nasal area (rhinophyma), congestive centrofacial erythema (Photo: Albanova V.I.)

- Gnathophyma (chin)
- Metophyma (forehead)
- Blepharophyma (eyelids)
- Otophyma (earlobe)

The phymatous form is characterized by hypervascularization, telangiectasias, and sebaceous hyperplasia, while midface redness and telangiectasias may not be present (**Table I-2-4**).

Table I-2-4. Severity of the phymatous rosacea

MILD	MODERATE	SEVERE
• Mild erythema • Minor swelling • Enlarged orifices of the pilosebaceous follicle (pores)	• Moderate erythema • Moderate swelling and enlargement of the nose • Moderate hyperplasia of the nasal soft tissue	• Severe erythema • A pronounced enlargement of the nose • Significant overgrowth of the nasal soft tissue

Ophthalmorosacea

Ophthalmorosacea (synonyms: eye rosacea, ocular rosacea, ophthalmorosacea) may precede or accompany skin lesions (**Fig. I-2-7**). Flashes of eyelid and conjunctival redness are independent of the activity or severity of the facial lesions and may occur independently of facial flare-ups. High sensitivity to light, the sensation of "sand" in the eyes, blurred vision, and reactions to cosmetics and medications are the main characteristics (**Table I-2-5**).

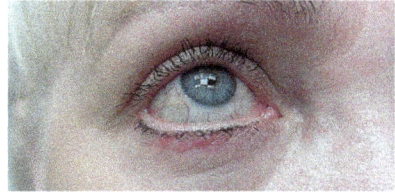

Figure I-2-7. Ophthalmorosacea: redness and swelling of eyelids, telangiectasias (Photo: Albanova V.I.)

Table I-2-5. Severity of the ophthalmorosacea

MILD	MODERATE	SEVERE
• Minor dryness/itching • Minor conjunctival injection	• Burning/tingling • Blepharitis, chalazion or hordeolum • Moderate conjunctival injection	• Pain • Fear of light • Severe blepharitis, episcleritis • Conjunctival and pericorneal injection

2.2.3. Clinical manifestation of rosacea according to the 2017 classification

As mentioned above, the classification based on the phenotypic approach allows the diagnosis and treatment of rosacea according to the characteristic features of the patient's disease based on pre-defined "narrow" subtypes, thereby individualizing care and optimizing treatment outcomes.

In 2019, the US National Rosacea Community's classification of specialists was supplemented by the consensus of the global ROSacea COnsensus (ROSCO) project, which included an international panel of expert dermatologists and ophthalmologists from Europe, North America, and South America, Africa, and Asia (Gallo R. et al., 2018; Schaller M. et al., 2020). **Table I-2-6** summarizes the results reported by these two groups.

Table I-2-6. Cutaneous features of rosacea according to the consensus of the US National Rosacea Community (2017) and ROSCO (2019) (Gallo R. et al., 2018; Schaller M. et al., 2020).

SYMPTOM	CLINICAL MANIFESTATION
Diagnostic signs	
Persistent erythema	• Persistent centrofacial erythema is a persistent reddening of the skin of the central part of the face, clearly visible in skin phototype I–IV • In darker phototypes (V and VI), erythema can be difficult to detect visually (this is also why people with darker skin are less likely to be diagnosed with rosacea, although they also suffer from this pathology) • Although the redness is persistent, it may occasionally increase in response to triggers
Phymatous skin changes	• Thickening of the facial skin due to fibrosis and/or sebaceous gland hyperplasia • The nose is most severely affected, and its tissues can become very overgrown, taking on an ugly appearance (rhinophyma)
Key features	
Hot flashes/transient erythema	• Temporary increase in redness of the central part of the face, which may include a sensation of warmth, heat, burning, and/or pain • Can last a few seconds to minutes
Papules and pustules	• Red papules and pustules located predominantly in the centrofacial area • Large and deep elements may appear
Telangiectasias	• Visible vessels in the centrofacial area, which may be obscured in people with skin phototype V and VI, but are detected by dermatoscopy
Secondary attributes	
Burning	• Uncomfortable or painful sensation of heat, usually in the centrofacial region
Tingling sensation	• Uncomfortable or painful acute tingling sensation, usually in the centrofacial region
Edema	• Localized facial edema, which may be soft or firm (without pitting), and may be self-limiting in duration or permanent
Feeling of dry skin	• The skin of the centrofacial zone is rough to the touch • May be accompanied by peeling, burning, or tingling sensations

The 2017 guidelines do not provide a standardized protocol for assessing the severity of specific forms of rosacea in a phenotypic approach. Thus, the use appropriate scales to evaluate each of the signs is advised. However, the 2019 recommendations advocate focus on the following parameters:

- **Burning:** duration, frequency, intensity, degree (areas involved), associations with hot flashes, triggers, and lifestyle
- **Tingling:** duration, frequency, intensity, degree (areas involved), triggers, characterization of the sensation, and lifestyle
- **Edema:** duration, frequency, degree of swelling, extent of involvement (areas involved), diurnal variation, and lifestyle
- **Dry skin:** duration, frequency, intensity, extent of lesions (areas involved), itching, roughness, flaking, how often moisturizers should be applied, and lifestyle

Symptoms of the ocular form are described separately (**Table I-2-7**). Lesions involve the skin in the eye area and may extend to the eye's mucous membranes and even the iris. **Ophthalmorosacea** is relatively independent and may precede or accompany cutaneous lesions.

Table I-2-7. Ocular symptoms of rosacea according to the consensus of the US National Rosacea Community (2017) and ROSCO (2019) (Gallo R. et al., 2018; Schaller M. et al., 2020)

SYMPTOM	CLINICAL MANIFESTATION
Telangiectasias along the eyelid margin	The vessels at the edges of the eyelids are visible. May be difficult to detect with the naked eye in people with darker skin phototypes (V and VI)
Blepharitis	Inflammation of the eyelid margin, typically resulting from meibomian gland dysfunction
Keratitis	Inflammation of the cornea, which can lead to defects and, in the most severe cases, loss of vision
Conjunctivitis	Inflammation of the mucous membranes lining the inner surface of the eyelids and bulbar conjunctiva. Usually associated with conjunctival injection or vascular occlusion and conjunctival edema
Anterior uveitis	Inflammation of the iris and/or ciliary body

2.2.4. Specific forms of rosacea

Rosacea granulomatosa

The rashes are localized mainly in the periorbital or perioral areas. They are represented by hemispherical or flat reddish-brown papules 2–4 mm in diameter, with smooth, shiny surfaces, sharp borders, and rounded outlines. In some cases, the papules form a bumpy surface, tightly adhering to each other (**Fig. I-2-8**). Diascopy often reveals yellow-brown spots, which may lead to their misinterpretation as a sign of tuberculosis — "apple jelly."

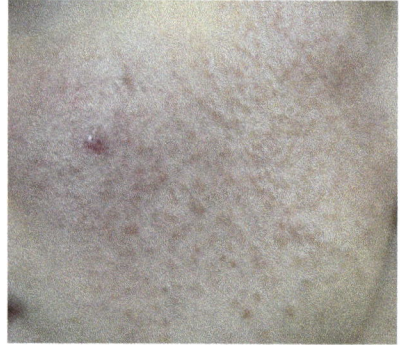

Figure I-2-8. Rosacea granulomatosa

Rosacea conglobata

In the clinical picture, in addition to hyperemia, papules, pustules, and telangiectasias, there are nodular elements of a bluish-red or brownish-red color that are spherical in shape and 1.5–2 cm in diameter (**Fig. I-2-9**).

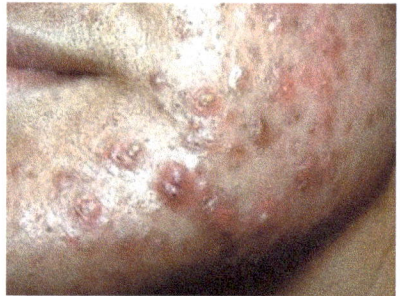

Figure I-2-9. Rosacea conglobata

Rosacea fulminans

Occurs suddenly, against the background of the general well-being of the body. Severe edema and scarlet or bluish-red erythema, papules and pustules, large nodes of hemispherical and spherical shape, often with fluctuation and brownish-yellow crusts on the surface are formed. a thick, lumpy conglomerate emerges due to the confluence of the nodules (**Fig. I-2-10**). Localized

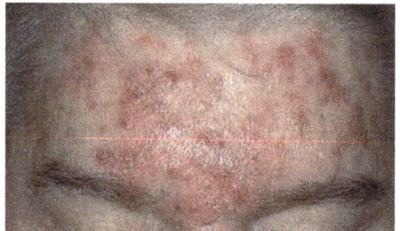

Figure I-2-10. Rosacea fulminans

soreness, burning, itching, and a feeling of tightness are the most common complaints. Typical rash localization sites are the forehead, cheeks, and chin.

Rosacea gram-negative

This is a complicative form of rosacea that emerges after long-term rosacea therapy with topical or systemic antibiotics (mainly of the tetracycline series) with primary action against gram-positive pathogens. This therapy leads to the selection of gram-negative pathogens. The clinical picture is characterized by pustular formations on newly formed or already existing extensive erythema (**Fig. I-2-11**). There is

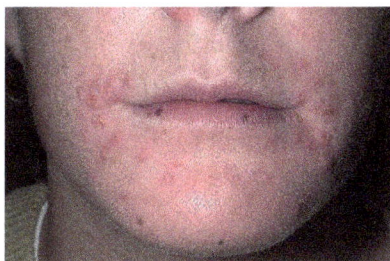

Figure I-2-11. Rosacea gram-negative

no clinical difference relative to rosacea papulopustulosa. However, since the treatment regimen differs, a distinction between rosacea gram-negative and rosacea papulopustulosa is necessary.

Chapter 3
Diagnostics

3.1. Diagnosis

As discussed in the previous chapter, rosacea is diagnosed based on the presence of specific clinical symptoms:

- According to the 2002 classification, the diagnostic criterion for rosacea is **persistent erythema in the central part of the face, existing for three months**.
- According to the 2017 classification, the diagnostic criterion is the presence of either **persistent erythema accompanied by phymatous changes** or **any two symptoms from the main features** (flashes/transient erythema, inflammatory papules and pustules, telangiectasia, ocular manifestations).

In both classifications, the remaining signs and symptoms are considered additional factors that determine the disease's severity and clinical form.

Therefore, to correctly identify all symptoms and features of the disease course, it is necessary to collect a detailed history and examine the patient. The anamnesis specifies the duration of complaints, their progression, localization, trigger factors for each sign, family history, and lifestyle habits.

Physical examination involves clarification of each sign's localization and degree of severity. The phymatous type is characterized by the presence of enlarged skin pores, skin thickening, and irregular bumpiness of the skin of the nose (rhinophyma), forehead (metaphyma), chin (gnathophyma), and auricles (otophyma), and less often eyelids (blepharophyma).

The use of laboratory and instrumental methods for diagnosing rosacea is usually not required, but may be necessary for differential diagnosis.

3.2. Differential diagnosis

Since rosacea is characterized by symptoms typical for many other skin diseases, errors in its diagnosis often occur, which leads to the prescription of ineffective therapy and, consequently, absence of symptom improvement and even progression of the disease. To prevent such situations, when the patient initially seeks professional help, it is necessary to carry out a complete **differential diagnosis**.

3.2.1. Erythematotelangiectatic rosacea

The differential diagnosis of erythematotelangiectatic rosacea should be made with the following diseases and conditions:
- Chronic photodamage
- Morbihan disease
- Steroid dermatitis
- Contact dermatitis
- Seborrheic dermatitis
- Early manifestations of cutaneous and systemic lupus erythematosus
- Flash syndrome (Asian red-face syndrome)
- Niacin-related redness flare-ups

Chronic photodamage is the closest clinical presentation to this rosacea form (**Table I-3-1**). As sun exposure is a trigger factor for both pathologies, in some cases, they may coexist.

Table I-3-1. Differential diagnosis of erythematotelangiectatic rosacea and chronic photodamage

ERYTHEMATOTELANGIECTATIC ROSACEA	CHRONIC PHOTODAMAGE
Centrofacial redness	Diffuse redness involving the lateral areas of the face and neck
No poikiloderma	Poikiloderma
Erythema flare-up aggravation	No flashes

Many experts consider **Morbihan disease** as a special form of rosacea (so-called solid facial edema in rosacea). Solid erythema and edema slowly spread from the forehead to the eyelids, then to the cheeks, without any subjective sensations (**Fig. I-3-1**). Solid edema and the clinical manifestations (spreading from the forehead) make distinguishing between the two diseases possible.

Steroid dermatitis due to long-term use of systemic or topical glucocorticosteroids is so similar to rosacea that it is often called steroid rosacea (or steroid-induced rosacea). Sometimes three months is enough to develop steroid dermatitis, but it may require up to 10 years. Diffuse redness, withdrawal syndrome, burning or itching, dry skin, telangiectasia, and papulopustular rashes are the main characteristics of this condition, assisting in the differential diagnosis (**Table I-3-2**).

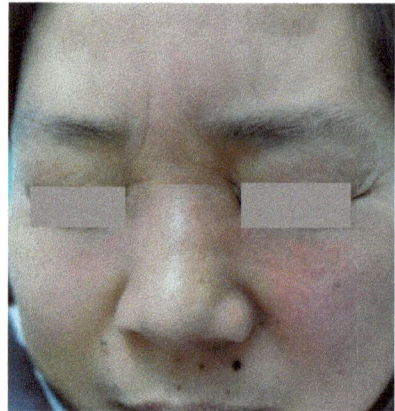

Figure I-3-1. Morbihan disease: non-pitting edema and erythema of the upper two-thirds of the face (adapted from Zhou L.F., Lu R., 2022)

Table I-3-2. Differential diagnosis of erythematotelangiectatic rosacea and steroid dermatitis

ERYTHEMATOTELANGIECTATIC ROSACEA	STEROID DERMATITIS
Centrofacial location	Diffuse localization (but may be centro-facial)
Erythema flare-ups	No flashes
Not related to glucocorticosteroids	History of long-term treatment with glucocorticosteroids
Mostly affects those aged 30–60 years	Mostly found in those aged 20–40 years
Blepharitis and conjunctival hyperemia frequently present	Rarely, the eyes are involved

In **seborrheic dermatitis**, the location of erythemato-squamous rashes in the middle part of the face and the frequent presence of papules and pustules due to concomitant acne may cause differential diagnostic difficulties. The medical history (the onset of the disease with increased skin oiliness, improvement in summer, the absence of erythema flare-ups), and the clinical picture (uneven skin, sebaceous scales in seborrheic dermatitis, smooth skin, and telangiectasias in rosacea) helps in making a distinction between this condition and rosacea.

Flash syndrome occurs mainly in Asians (Koreans, Chinese, and Japanese in particular, hence the commonly used alternative name — Asian red-face syndrome) after consuming even a tiny amount of alcohol. Redness is accompanied by tachycardia, increased blood pressure, and skin temperature. Acetaldehyde accumulates in the body, due to a mutation in the *ALDH2* gene (common in those of Asian descent) responsible for encoding the synthesis of the enzyme acetaldehyde dehydrogenase, which usually breaks down acetaldehyde, the main product of ethanol metabolism.

Taking **niacin** or **niacinamide** can cause hyperemia of the skin and upper half of the trunk, paresthesias, dizziness, blood flushes to the face, and arrhythmia.

3.2.2. Rosacea papulopustulosa

In the differential diagnosis of the rosacea papulopustulosa the following diseases should be considered:
- Papulopustular acne
- Demodicosis
- Perioral dermatitis

Acne vulgaris
First, rosacea must be distinguished from acne vulgaris. As the clinical pictures of these diseases are similar (**Fig. I-3-2**, **Table I-3-3**), rosacea was called *pink acne* for a long time, which created additional confusion. Even now, it can be challenging to differentiate the two

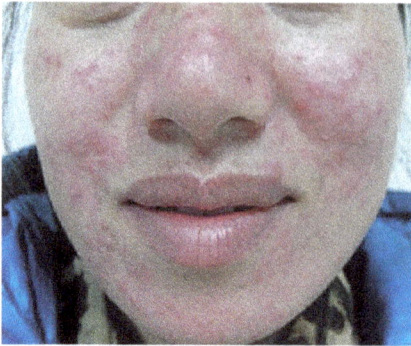

Papulopustular rosacea:
typical lesions such as erythema, papules, and pustules on the face

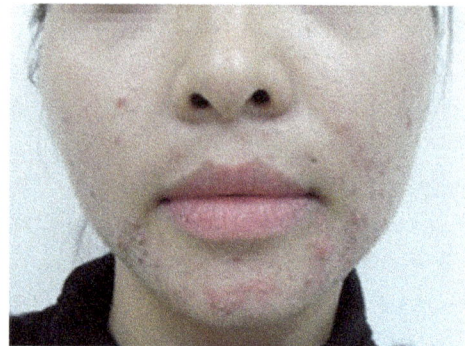

Acne vulgaris:
typical lesions such as comedones, papules, and pustules on the face

Figure I-3-2. Papulopustular rosacea *vs.* acne vulgaris (adapted from Zhou M. et al., 2016)

conditions, especially if the erythema is minimal. The differential diagnosis is also problematic when patients are affected by both diseases simultaneously.

Table I-3-3. Papulopustular rosacea *vs.* acne vulgaris

PAPULOPUSTULAR ROSACEA	ACNE VULGARIS
Beginning in adulthood (30–60 years)	Onset during puberty
Not related to hormonal influences	Related to hormonal influence (aggravation due to menstruation, pregnancy)
No comedones	Open and closed comedones
Only the face is affected	Presence of rashes on the chest and back
Erythema flare-ups	No flashes
Erythema centrofacialis, telangiectasia	No erythema or telangiectasia
Exacerbation by insolation	Improvement with insolation
No scarring	Post-acne scars are common
Worsening with age	Improvement with age
Blepharitis and conjunctival hyperemia frequently present	No eye involvement

Perioral dermatitis

Perioral dermatitis is another rosacea-like disease, but its diagnosis should not cause difficulties (**Table I-3-4**). Papules around the mouth and nostrils are characterized by background redness and a pale red border (**Fig. I-3-3**).

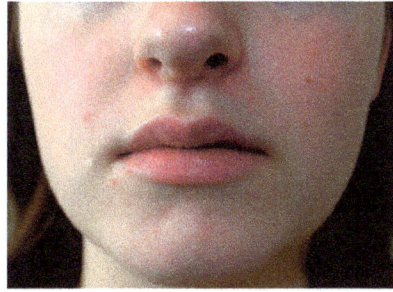

Figure I-3-3. Perioral dermatitis (Image by J. Köhle, Wikipedia)

Table I-3-4. Papulopustular rosacea *vs.* perioral dermatitis

PAPULOPUSTULAR ROSACEA	PERIORAL DERMATITIS
Predominantly centrofacial location of rashes	Perioral location
Centrofacial erythema, erythema flares, telangiectasia	No centrofacial erythema, no flare-ups, and no telangiectasia
Large pink-red colored papules and pustules	Small pink or skin-colored papules, with papules and pustules in the perioral area that tend to merge, absence near the red border of the lips
Multiple localization sites	One localization sites
Age of onset: 30–60 years	Age of onset: 20–40 years
Often involving blepharitis and conjunctival hyperemia	Usually no eye involvement

Demodicosis

Demodicosis is another type of dermatosis that can be confused with rosacea. The contribution of *Demodex* mites to the pathogenesis of rosacea has been established, but other previously discussed factors are also necessary for developing this disease. Therefore, demodicosis can be present without rosacea, just as patients can develop rosacea without an overabundance of *Demodex* mites on their skin.

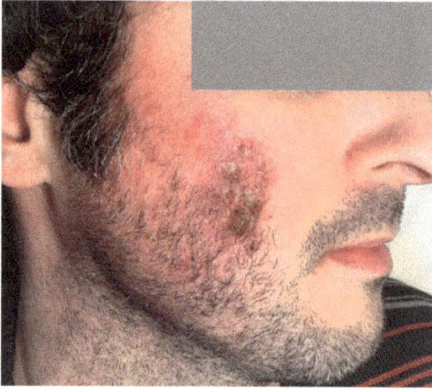

Demodicosis folliculitis: erythematous spots, scaling follicular papules on the surface, pustules on the face and scalp, dry, flaky, rough skin, lesions may be unilateral (Image by Casas M.N. et al., 2020)

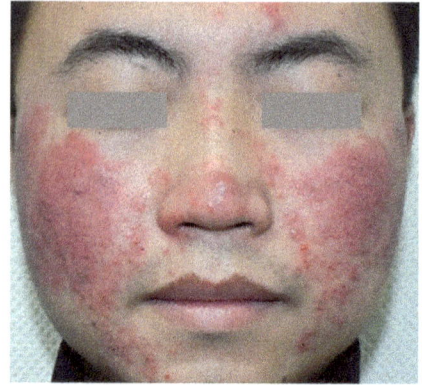

Papulopustular demodicosis: rashes (predominantly perioral and periorbital), solid erythema, often symmetrical (Image by Ran Yuping et al., Wikipedia)

Figure I-3-4. Demodicosis

There are two forms of demodicosis (**Fig. I-3-4**). *Demodicosis folliculitis* is characterized by erythematous patches, papules with scales, and pustules on the face and scalp. Dry, flaky, rough skin is noted, and the lesion may be unilateral. In the **papulopustular form**, rashes are predominantly around the eyes and mouth and occur symmetrically.

Localization, late onset of the disease (after 30 years of age), lack of association with hormonal influences, and characteristic subjective sensations indicate demodicosis (**Table I-3-5**).

Table I-3-5. Papulopustular rosacea *vs.* demodicosis

PAPULOPUSTULAR ROSACEA	DEMODICOSIS
Rashes in the central area of the face	Rashes around the mouth and eyes
No rashes on the scalp	Rashes on the skin of the scalp frequently present
Erythema is symmetrical, rashes are also more often located on both sides of the face	There may be a unilateral lesion (for demodectic folliculitis)
Centrofacial erythema	Erythematous spots

Chapter 4
Impact of lifestyle on rosacea treatment

As rosacea is a progressive disease, it is impossible to talk about a full recovery. In addition, skin hypersensitivity and frequent medication and skincare product intolerance are the main obstacles to the identification and application of the most effective treatment methods. As Albert Kligman, a famous American dermatologist, said in 2003: "Rosacea is a highly distressing, psychologically debilitating, lifelong disease."

Therefore, the primary aim of any therapy is to achieve remission, slow the disease progression, and improve patients' quality of life. This goal is attainable, as ample evidence demonstrates that many methods can provide relief, and encouraging results can be achieved by combining various medical, cosmetic, and physiotherapy methods (Del Rosso J.Q. et al., 2014; Weinkle A.P. et al., 2015). Moreover, the understanding of rosacea pathogenesis has significantly improved in recent years, which opens new perspectives.

Currently utilized approaches to rosacea therapy and control include:

- Lifestyle adjustments
- Medication assistance
- Cosmetic skincare
- Physiotherapy
- Nutrition

These approaches work only in combination, as an appropriate lifestyle is the basis for successful treatment. Rosacea patients must change their lifestyle significantly, as many simple actions for healthy people can exacerbate the disease. Thus, the participants of the *Rosacea: Beyond the Visible* study discussed in Chapter 1 reported having to avoid:

- Sun exposure (50%)
- Alcoholic beverages (33%)
- Spicy food (26%)
- Bath or sauna (25%)
- Hot weather (24%)
- Makeup (21%)
- Cosmetic products (21%)
- Cold weather (19%)
- Social contact (17%)
- Public pools (15%)
- Sports activities (15%)
- Hot food (13%)
- Computer use (7%)
- Gardening (6%)
- Long reads (5%)
- Car driving (4%)
- Other activities (1%)

However, 14% of those surveyed did not report any limitations in their everyday activity range or level.

As evident from the list presented above, these changes are individualized, and to identify them, it is necessary to interview the patient thoroughly, perhaps asking them to keep a lifestyle diary (just like a food diary and a diary of cosmetic use) to identify specific triggers. This approach will help minimize the activity restrictions to the essentials.

Rosacea patients are generally advised to avoid sun exposure, extreme temperatures, baths, saunas, hot baths and showers, warming procedures, intensive physical labor, and sports exercises. The good news is that, with proper treatment and achieved remission, many of these pleasures of life become possible, albeit in moderation.

Before proceeding to therapy, we note that **at the heart of any therapeutic measures for treating rosacea is adequate daily skincare and the use of sunscreen.**

Chapter 5
Medication treatment

5.1. Drugs

The following groups of medications are currently used to treat rosacea: kallikrein-5 inhibitors, vasoconstrictor drugs, antibacterial drugs, antiprotozoal and antiparasitic drugs, and retinoids.

Kallikrein-5 inhibitors

Topical: gel with azelaic acid 15% (Skinoren). Azelaic acid has moderate anti-inflammatory, antioxidant, antimicrobial, and anti-keratinizing effects and regulates sebum lipid production in sebocytes, reducing the production of long-chain fatty acids.

Systemic: doxycycline (Unidox solutab). It is believed that the primary active mechanism of doxycycline in rosacea is anti-inflammatory rather than antimicrobial (Yentzer B.A., Fleischer A.B., 2010).

Vasoconstrictor drugs

The sympathetic nervous system regulates the maintenance of vascular tone via the nerve fibers woven into the smooth muscle wall of the blood vessel. Its action is realized through different types of adrenoreceptors. Topical vasoconstrictors, being α-adrenergic receptor agonists, help counteract rosacea-related vascular dysfunction.

The drug of choice is 0.33% brimonidine tartrate gel. Brimonidine has affinity primarily to α_2-adrenergic receptors, acting much less significantly on α_1-adrenic receptors, i.e., it is a highly selective agonist of α_2-adrenergic receptors. Oxymetazoline 1% solution can be used to "target" α_1-adrenergic receptors (Del Rosso J.Q. et al., 2014).

In addition to vasoconstriction, both compounds have anti-inflammatory effects (Beck-Speier I. et al., 2009; Jackson J.M. et al., 2015; Okwundu N. et al., 2019).

Antibacterial drugs
Systemic: erythromycin, azithromycin, and clarithromycin, which can be prescribed in cases of doxycycline intolerance.
Topical: Dalacin gel, Zerkalin solution, Fucidin cream, Basiron AC gel at 5% and 2.5% concentration.

Antiprotozoal and antiparasitic drugs
Systemic: metronidazole, ornidazole. Metronidazole is also believed to have anti-inflammatory and antioxidant effects (Tan J. et al., 2017).
Topical: ivermectin (Ivermectin cream), metronidazole formulations (Metrogyl gel, Rozex cream, Rozamet cream). Ivermectin is an antiparasitic drug that has a pronounced anti-inflammatory effect when applied topically. It is also active against *Demodex* mites.

Retinoids
Systemic: isotretinoin in low doses (0.3 mg/kg/day) or microdoses (0.03–0.17 mg/kg/day) (Roaccutane, Sotret, Acnecutan), retinol palmitate. Low doses of isotretinoin are thought to inhibit phymatous changes due to its anti-inflammatory activity and a reduction in sebum.
Topical: isotretinoin (retinoic acid ointment 0.05% and 0.1%), adapalene (Differin gel and cream, Klenzit gel, Adaclean cream).

The following medicines may also be prescribed:
- Zinc preparations: Zincteral pills, Zinkit pills
- Sedatives: tinctures of valerian, peony, motherwort
- Vegetotropic agents: Valocordin drops
- Hyposensitizing agents: calcium gluconate, calcium glycerophosphate, sodium thiosulfate
- Calcineurin inhibitors: Elidel cream, Protopic ointment
- Anti-inflammatory and barrier-strengthening agents: niacinamide, vitamins C and E

5.2. Recommended administration regimen

Treatment guidelines for rosacea according to the 2019 ROSCO consensus are provided in **Table I-5-1** (Schaller M. et al., 2020).

Table I-5-1. Treatment guidelines for rosacea according to the 2019 ROSCO consensus (Schaller M. et al., 2020)

FIRST-LINE THERAPY	TRANSIENT ERYTHEMA (FLARE-UPS)			PERSISTENT ERYTHEMA			PAPULES, PUSTULES			TELANGIECTASIAS			INFLAMMATORY PHYMATOUS CHANGES			NON-INFLAMMATORY PHYMATOUS CHANGES		
	1	2	3	1	2	3	1	2	3	1	2	3	1	2	3	1	2	3
Cosmetic products (sun protection and skincare)	+	+	+	+	+	+	+	+	+	+	+	+	+	+	+	+	+	+
Topical agents																		
Adrenergic receptor agonists*	+	+	+	+	+	+												
Azelaic acid							+	+										
Ivermectin							+	+	+									
Metronidazole							+	+										
β-blockers*	+	+	+															
Doxycycline**							+	+	+				+	+	+			
Isotretinoin									+				+	+	+			
Energy-based therapy																		
Electrosurgery										+	+	+						
IPL				+	+	+				+	+	+						
Vascular lasers				+	+	+				+	+	+						
Surgery																+	+	+

1 — mild; 2 — moderate; 3 — severe.

* There is little evidence supporting the use of topical α-adrenergic modulating agents or orally administrated β-blockers (nadolol and propranolol) for the treatment of hot flashes/transient erythema (Logger J.G.M. et al., 2020). However, the clinical experience of the experts making the recommendations suggests that they may be effective in some patients.

** The U.S. Food and Drug Administration (FDA) has approved using only a low dose (≤ 40 mg) of doxycycline for treating rosacea. It is believed that, in these quantities, doxycycline realizes its anti-inflammatory effects but not antibacterial ones. At the same time, studies have shown comparable rosacea treatment results with 100 mg and 40 mg dosages. In connection with the worldwide problem of antibiotic resistance development, the ability to achieve the desired effects with low doses of drugs that do not have bacteriostatic action is of particular importance.

EPSOLY® cream (Galderma) with encapsulated benzoyl peroxide 5% has received U.S. Food and Drug Administration (FDA) approval for treating mild to moderate papulopustular rosacea. The action of benzoyl peroxide is due to the release of atomic oxygen. In cosmetic dermatology, benzoyl peroxide is used for acne therapy. It possesses keratolytic, brightening, antibacterial, and anti-inflammatory properties, but being a peroxide, it is highly irritating to the skin. Because of this side-effect, benzoyl peroxide has not been used in rosacea, as it is a highly sensitive skin condition, although its properties are potentially beneficial. In the FDA-approved drug, benzoyl peroxide is "hidden" in microcapsules made of porous silicon dioxide. The slow migration of the benzoyl peroxide from the microcapsules allows for a metered delivery to the skin. At the same time, the capsule walls reduce the ability of benzoyl peroxide to cause severe oxidation, preventing associated irritation.

As for the treatment of ophthalmorosacea, since this book is intended for skincare practitioners, we will not touch upon it — it is the responsibility of ophthalmologists. a skincare specialist must be able to suspect these changes (see Part I, section 2.2) and refer the patient to an ophthalmologist.

Chapter 6
Cosmetic care

Proper cosmetic care is the basis of any therapeutic measure. The rosacea skincare program is aimed at:

- Facial cleansing
- Reducing existing irritation and inflammation
- Restoration of the epidermal barrier, moisturizing
- Strengthening of vessel walls and shrinkage of dilated capillaries
- Maintaining a healthy microbiome
- Camouflaging redness with special makeup products
- Protection, especially against UV radiation and pollution

Rosacea can affect the skin with any level of sebum production (sebum deficiency, as well as normal or excessive sebum production) and hydration (dry or sufficiently moisturized). Accordingly, preparations for cleansing and care should be selected individually and **strictly according to the skin condition and type**. However, there are general recommendations for all skin types, so before moving onto specific approaches, let's dwell on general expert advice on choosing skincare products.

6.1. Selecting cosmetic products

Regular gentle skincare and special decorative cosmetics will help the rosacea patient look and feel better, but only if they adhere to the critical rule: **avoid irritation**. The label "for sensitive skin" or "for skin with rosacea" can serve as a guide when choosing cosmetics, although it is not a 100% guarantee that no irritation will occur.

In a study involving 1,066 patients initiated by the US National Rosacea Society, many patients reported having reactions to cosmetics:

41% of participants complained of a general worsening of skin condition when using certain cosmetics, and 21% said that certain products triggered rosacea exacerbation.

To avoid adverse reactions and irritation, experts recommend adhering to the following rules when choosing skincare products and decorative cosmetics.

1. **Make sure the ingredient list is free of potential irritants and traumatizing agents.** In a study conducted by the US National Rosacea Society, the most common irritation triggers cited by patients were substances such as:
   - Alcohol (66%)
   - Witch hazel extract (30%)
   - Fragrances (30%)
   - Menthol (21%)
   - Mint (14%)
   - Eucalyptus essential oil (13%)

   Most respondents also indicated that they avoided tightening agents, exfoliating agents, and other ingredients potentially harmful to sensitive skin.

2. **Choose products that do not contain fragrances (synthetic fragrances or natural essential oils).** According to the American Academy of Dermatology, "fragrances are more likely to cause contact dermatitis than other substances." Skin is a large target for exogenous allergens, which can compromise the already weak barrier of sensitive skin. Accordingly, their use increases the risk of irritation. Please note that the label "allergy tested" should not be confused with "hypoallergenic" which is not strictly defined in cosmetic legislation.

3. **A new product should be tested first.** Before applying a new product to your face, you should test it on another part of your body, such as your neck. If there is an unwanted reaction, it should not be used. It is necessary to carefully read and remember the ingredients in its composition. Substances provoking hot flashes and rosacea aggravation differ from person to person, so it is essential to make an individual list of "forbidden" substances.

4. **If possible, minimize the number of cosmetic products used.** It is desirable to choose multifunctional products, thus reducing their total number. The fewer ingredients they contain, the better.

Substances that can provoke and aggravate rosacea:
- Synthetic fragrances
- Essential oils (all of them without exception)
- Extracts of strongly aromatic plants such as cinnamon, rosemary, lavender, rose, etc.
- Extracts of lemon, lime, mint, pineapple, cedar
- Menthol and its derivatives
- Alcohol (the ingredient list indicates SD alcohol or Alcohol denatured)
- Hazelnut extract
- Salts of fatty acids (natural soap), sodium lauryl sulfate, sodium laureth sulfate, and other high-foaming surfactants

Products to be avoided:
- Natural bar soaps
- Abrasive scrubs
- Alcohol-containing cleansers
- Alcohol- and fragrance-containing toners
- Acid peels
- Brushes

6.2. Skin cleansing

Gentle cleansing is an essential step of the rosacea skincare routine. The face should be washed at least twice a day to remove excess sebum, impurities, microorganisms, and residues of cosmetics and decorative cosmetics.

When cleansing, **never use scrubs, sponges, or any mechanical means that may traumatize the skin**. The cleanser should be applied only with fingertips through gentle circular movements, without rubbing or stretching the skin.

6.2.1. Cleansers

Different products can be used to clean rosacea-affected skin, provided no risky substances exist. Substances that can be applied to healthy skin without any complications may aggravate rosacea, as if the epidermal barrier is damaged, they cause irritation, inflammation, and unpleasant sensation.

Surfactants are potentially harmful cosmetic ingredients. Their molecules are elongated and polar. Most of the molecule is the elongated hydrophobic part, which avoids contact with water. Attached to it at one end is a relatively small hydrophilic group, which is usually charged and faces toward water. Surfactants localize at the interface of immiscible phases, such as oil and water, and cause a decrease in the surface tension between them.

Surfactants dissociating in water to form ions are called **ionic**. There are two ionic surfactants: **cationic** (dissociate in cations, which are positively charged ions) and **anionic** (dissociate in anions, i.e., negatively charged ions). Non-dissociating surfactants are **non-ionic**. **Amphoteric (zwitterionic)** surfactants contain two functional groups. Depending on the pH, these surfactants can exist in an anionic, cationic, or non-ionic state.

The dermatological properties of surfactants depend on the charge: cationic surfactants **(+)** are more irritating to the skin than anionic surfactants **(–)**, and anionic surfactants are more irritating than non-ionic surfactants **(0)**. Thus, the intensity of skin irritation follows the order **(+) > (–) > (0)** making the non-ionic surfactants the safest.

Some of the gentle non-ionic surfactants suitable for rosacea-affected skin are given below:

- Alkanolamides
- Alkyl glycosides
- Alkylamines
- Alkylated amino acids
- Cocamidopropyl betaine
- Coco amino propionic acid
- Poloxamers
- Polyoxyethylated fatty acids
- Polyoxyethylated sorbitol esters

- Sodium cocoafopropionate
- Sodium lauraminopropionate
- Sodium lauroamoacetate

Surfactants are contraindicated for hypersensitive skin with impaired barrier properties, as they can penetrate the lipid barrier and embed themselves in it, causing further damage. Therefore, surfactant-free **micellar solutions** are recommended instead of traditional liquid or bar soap. Micellar solution is a suspension of lipid-composed micelles in water (**Fig. I-6-1**). When applied to the skin, the lipids embed into the fatty plaques on the skin surface and crush them. While micellar solutions will never be as effective as soap as cleansers due to the absence of surfactants, they are preferred for cleaning very sensitive skin.

People with rosacea can also use cleansing milk based on a soft and light emulsion. It is worth noting that milk also contains surfactants, as they are always present even in the most diluted emulsions. But if the sensitive skin is quite heavily polluted, it is better to wipe it with milk and reserve the micellar solution for cleansing not very polluted skin.

Note: **Regardless of the damaged skin's contamination, people with rosacea cannot use traditional soap with fatty acid salts as surfactants and pH over 9**. Nonetheless, **syndets** (= **syn**thetic **de**tergents) are still preferable, as these liquid or bar cleansing products have a pH of 5.6–6.5.

Today, new cleansing products that also contain surfactants are increasingly being brought to the cosmetics market, but they are different from traditional surfactants, and their number is still relatively low. Such gentle surfactants make bringing the pH to the desired values

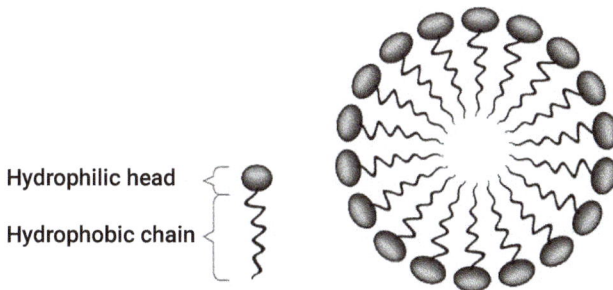

Hydrophilic head
Hydrophobic chain

Figure I-6-1. Micelle structure

possible without harming the epidermal barrier. The physiological pH of human skin is 4.5–5.5, so if people with rosacea need soap for heavily soiled skin, they should use syndets. They can look like both solid and liquid soaps — the main thing is that the pH is balanced.

6.2.2. Choosing a cleaning product

The choice of cleanser for rosacea-affected skin depends on the sebum production. As mentioned earlier, the disease can affect the facial skin at any level of sebum production. In sebum excess, the choice should fall on a non-soap cleanser free of fatty acid salts (no more than 10% of these substances are allowed). For those with insufficient sebum, light emulsion (cosmetic milk) containing emollients is recommended. In all cases, without exception, the pH of the cleanser should be slightly acidic and should correspond to the physiological pH of the skin surface (i.e., not exceeding 5.5).

Normal sebum production
Cosmetic milk for damaged skin or a micellar solution can be used for skin with normal or slightly reduced sebum production. However, while cosmetic milk can be removed with sponges, **micellar solutions must be rinsed off the skin!** The soft cleansing base of emulsions is usually enriched with soothing plant extracts (calendula, rose, mallow), and softening components (apricot kernel oil, glycerin). Soap-free emulsions have a physiological pH of about 5.5 and a light gel-like texture.

Low sebum production
For dry low-sebum skin, it is advisable to use mild soap-free cleansers based on micellar solutions or light emulsion (cosmetic milk), free from traditional surfactants and alcohol, with soothing substances (plant extracts of chamomile, arnica, calendula, aloe, etc.). a creamy, low-foaming, soap-free cleanser may be the best choice, as it both cleanses and moisturizes the skin.

Sebum overproduction (oily skin)
Those with oily skin (i.e., with excessive sebum production) should choose a dermatologically mild soap, preferably syndet. It can be in

solid or liquid form, but the main thing is that it does not contain fatty acid salts, and its water solution has a pH of about 5.5. It should not be rubbed onto the skin and left on the face for long. If the dirt is not completely removed the first time, it is better to soap several times and rinse thoroughly with warm water after each application.

Salicylic and enzymatic exfoliating products can be used for oily, flaking skin to loosen the *stratum corneum* and promote exfoliation. Still, they should be used carefully.

To summarize, mild products should be used for cleansing rosacea-affected skin, preferably non-foaming cream or micellar products that will also support the skin's natural protective functions.

6.2.3. Cleansing routine

To minimize skin irritation, people with rosacea should follow this gentle, step-by-step cleansing routine recommended by the US National Rosacea Society (www.rosacea.org):

1. Using your fingertips, wash the skin with a cleanser suitable for your skin type. Avoid using an abrasive washcloth or sponge, which may irritate.
2. Rinse away the cleanser with lukewarm water, as hot or cold water may cause flushing or irritation. If your face is irritated by water at any temperature, try using a soothing cream cleanser you can simply take off.
3. Gently blot your face dry with a thick-pile cotton towel. Don't rub your skin, as this may cause irritation.
4. Since stinging most often occurs on damp skin, wait 30 minutes for the face to dry completely before applying topical medication. Slowly reduce the drying time until you find the least time your skin needs to avoid a stinging sensation.
5. After applying topical medication, wait 5–10 minutes before applying moisturizer, sunscreen, or makeup.
6. If you have ocular rosacea, follow your ophthalmologist's directions for eyelid scrubbing and medication.

In contact with water, the skin's barrier properties are further weakened, and the permeability to external agents increases. Serious consideration should thus be given to whether the skin needs more active ingredients in its deeper layers, whether this will increase the likelihood of more rapid development of undesirable adverse reactions, and whether the excipients will penetrate the skin, causing allergic reactions and other undesirable effects.

6.2.4. For men: shaving rosacea-affected skin

Shaving can further damage the skin. To minimize the risks, use an electric shaver and avoid alcohol-containing lotions and toners. After shaving, treat the skin with a nourishing balm or an individually selected moisturizer.

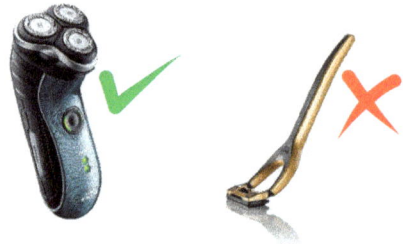

6.3. Restoring and strengthening the skin barrier

As the rosacea-affected skin has an impaired barrier, repairing and maintaining it is critical to rosacea management.

6.3.1. Hydrolipid mantle and surface pH

The hydrolipid mantle is constantly present on the skin, acting as a chemical barrier for foreign substances (**Fig. I-6-2**). The suppliers of its components are the sebaceous and

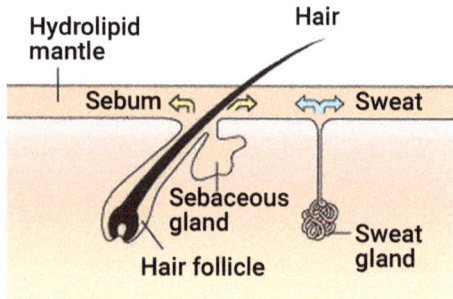

Figure I-6-2. Hydrolipid (acid) mantle of the skin

sweat glands, which release fatty and aqueous secretions onto the skin surface. The resulting mixture is an emulsion with both aqueous and oil phases. The average pH of the hydrolipid mantle varies from 4.5 to 5.8 depending on the location on the body. These are acidic values, so the hydrolipid mantle has another name — acid mantle.

The protective role of the acid mantle is that it keeps the skin microflora under control, preventing pathogenic microbes from colonizing the surface. Not all microorganisms can live in such an acidic environment, and only those that have adapted to these conditions remain on the skin's surface. But the skin, in turn, has adapted to such "guests." This peaceful coexistence is mainly possible due to the constant acidity of the mantle.

In rosacea, especially if sebum production is low, the skin is virtually devoid of the hydrolipid mantle. Since the sebum lipid balance is altered, it is much less able to cope with its functions.

Products that mimic the action of the acid mantle have a protective function because they take over its role (in other words, they restore the impaired barrier). These sebum analogs may contain natural sebum components, such as squalene. However, as the nature of the hydrolipid mantle disorder may differ, specific protective products should be selected, considering the skin condition and existing pathology.

For skin repair, **antioxidants** are universal components that are good in any situation. Oil-soluble antioxidants such as vitamin E and ubiquinone are suitable for strengthening the acid mantle. As for water-soluble antioxidants such as vitamin C and bioflavonoids, they impact even living cells, although this aspect is less relevant for rosacea-affected individuals. More importantly, they reduce the amount of oil-soluble antioxidants, so they should be used in tandem to extend the shelf life of the latter and protect them from oxidation. We will talk more about antioxidants in section 6.5.1.

Now, let's touch on the **pH** of cosmetic products. The pH (Latin *pondus hydrogenii* — hydrogen weight) is a measure of the activity of hydrogen ions in a solution, quantitatively expressing its acidity (or alkalinity). The numerical criterion for pH is a scale ranging from 0 to 14. a medium with a pH of 7 is neutral, one with a pH below 7 is acidic, and that with a pH exceeding 7 is alkaline. The pH scale is logarithmic, meaning that each division increases or decreases the acidity by a factor of 10 relative to the previous value. For example, a medium with a pH of 2 is 10 times more alkaline than a medium with a pH of 1. Accordingly, a medium with pH 3 will be 100 times more alkaline than that with pH 1.

In rosacea, alkalinization of the skin can occur due to changes in the balance of fatty acids in the sebum (Ní Raghallaigh S. et al., 2012). In this situation, the skin responds well to acidifying preparations. This approach is called **acid therapy**: products that remain in contact with the skin and are on the skin surface slightly acidify the hydrolipid mantle, thus maintaining a physiological pH. Therefore, slightly acidified products with a pH of about 4.5 can be recommended for rosacea management. More acidic products may cause burning. Modern preparations increasingly include polyhydroxy acids, such as lactobionic acid or gluconolactone, which not only acidify the skin but also moisturize it well (detailed information on this topic is available in the *Chemical Peeling in Cosmetic Dermatology & Skincare Practice* book).

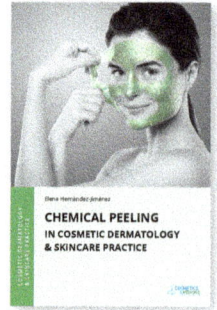

6.3.2. Strengthening the lipid barrier

When the epidermal barrier is restored, this condition should be maintained for as long as possible. The lipid barrier is built by lipids of three groups: ceramides, cholesterol, and free fatty acids. In normal conditions, their ratio is 1:1:1, i.e., the number of lipid molecules of each group in the lipid barrier is the same — such a mixture of substances is called equimolar. As we have already mentioned, this proportion is altered in the case of rosacea. It is **necessary to strengthen the barrier, increase its integrity, and provide a good antioxidant potential because all these aspects are weakened in rosacea-affected skin**.

The physiological constituents of intercellular lipids are **ceramides, cholesterol,** and **unsaturated fatty acids**. The skin responds very well to these substances, even though some patients may have oily skin. These physiological barrier lipids, unlike sebum lipids, do not remain on the surface but penetrate the *stratum corneum*, where they are incorporated into intercellular lipid bilayers.

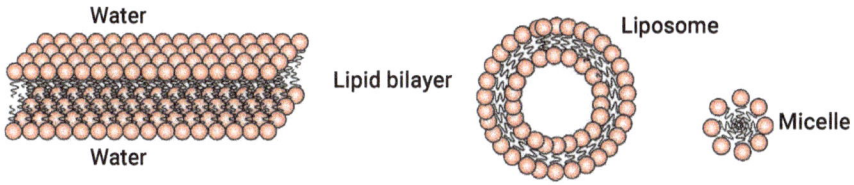

Figure I-6-3. Lipid structures: biological membranes, liposomes, and micelles

An equimolar mixture of ceramides/cholesterol/free fatty acids has been experimentally found to have the best restorative properties. It is no coincidence that lipids are among the most popular cosmetic ingredients. They can be included in formulations as individual molecules and structural entities such as liposomes and micelles (**Fig. I-6-3**). In addition to the traditional role assigned to lipids, such structures act as carriers or containers for other bioactive ingredients, stabilizing them and facilitating their penetration through the *stratum corneum*.

A popular technology in cosmetic production relies on using so-called multi-lamellar emulsions (MLE) based on phosphatidylcholine (lecithin). In MLE, tiny lipid droplets are stabilized not by conventional emulsifiers (surfactants) but by a network of bilayers like those that form the lipid barrier (**Fig. I-6-4**). "Preparations that structurally match the skin" is how these cosmetics are often described. They have excellent moisturizing and regenerating properties because they resemble the lipid barrier not only in composition but also in structure, which is especially important for dry low-sebum skin.

Oil- and water-soluble **antioxidants** are mandatory. As mentioned above, these antioxidants are needed to support the activity of oil-soluble "partners" and compensate for the insufficiency of the antioxidant system in rosacea (more details are given below).

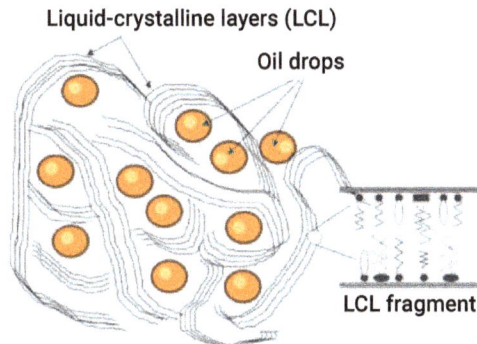

Figure I-6-4. Multi-lamellar emulsions (MLE)

6.3.3. Moisturizing the *stratum corneum*

Finally, rosacea-affected skin requires moisturization. While restoring the barrier function alone will help retain moisture, using a natural moisturizing factor (NMF) is recommended.

Hygroscopic "deep" moisturizers include the following topical substances:
- Amino acids
- Lactic acid, sodium lactate (in low concentrations)
- Sodium pyroglutamate
- Glycerin
- Sorbitol trioleate
- Glyceret-26
- Methyl gluceth-20
- Sorbic acid

Urea, one of the most well-known moisturizing factor components, is not recommended for use in rosacea because of its irritating potential.

Unlike high-molecular-weight compounds that remain on the skin surface, NMF components applied as a part of cosmetics penetrate the *stratum corneum* (but do not infiltrate deeper layers) and increase its water retention potential from the inside (that's why they say *deep moisturizing*). The moisturization that is felt in this way is usually not as pronounced and does not come on as quickly as the *wet compress* effect, but it lasts longer and is less dependent on the air humidity.

Separately, it should be said that **the use of occlusive products is not recommended** for patients with rosacea. These products contain petroleum jelly, mineral oil, lanolin, and solid oils (e.g., coconut oil) that "close" the skin and prevent transepidermal evaporation of water. Occlusion causes excess water to accumulate in the *stratum corneum*. The skin of rosacea patients may react negatively to such excessive moisturization, further increasing its permeability. Thus, there have been reports of rosacea exacerbations due to prolonged wearing of COVID-19 protection masks, a condition called mask-acea (Giacalone S. et al., 2021). Caution should also be exercised when using products containing high concentrations of shea butter, cocoa butter, mango butter, and highly concentrated silicones.

The modern cosmetic industry offers a wide range of moisturizers, differing in composition, chemical form, and mechanism of action. However, it should be remembered that not all of them are suitable for patients with rosacea.

1. Gel forms (including so-called serums) should be avoided as they can contribute to a feeling of tightness after drying. In oily skin, gels are acceptable, but only in humid climates.
2. Lamellar-based emulsions are preferred as they do not contain surfactants.
3. In the formulations, substances with soothing (niacinamide, allantoin, plant extracts of green tea, centella, boswellia, etc.) and softening (vegetable waxes, high-molecular-weight silicone oils) action are desirable.
4. Some formulations may contain green pigments that mask the red color of the skin.

6.4. Normalizing the skin microbiome

As we mentioned above, the microbial composition of the skin of rosacea patients differs from that of individuals with healthy skin. Although it is not completely clear whether these changes are secondary or primary, the change in the quantitative and qualitative composition of the hydrolipid mantle and local immune status, in any case, has serious consequences. Some previously dormant microorganisms begin to multiply actively and suppress their neighbors aggressively (van der Kolk T. et al., 2018).

A modern and promising strategy for combatting this issue is using cosmetics friendly to the skin microbiome. The cosmetic product mixes with its hydrolipidic mantle when applied to the skin. Together, they form a comfortable habitat for microorganisms. This is helped by special substances that have come into the cosmetics market from the food industry:

- **Probiotics:** live microorganisms that, when used in sufficient quantities, positively affect human health
- **Prebiotics:** selectively fermented media, the use of which has a positive effect on the skin ("feed" for bacteria)
- **Synbiotics:** an association of microorganisms with their nutrient medium

However, there is an important nuance when considering their topical application. Live microorganisms can be used as a part of food products to normalize intestinal microflora, but they cannot be introduced in topical products due to cosmetic legislation. One of the reasons for this restriction is that it is challenging to provide conditions for preserving beneficial microorganisms in the product without allowing the multiplication of "undesirable" microorganisms. One solution is introducing not bacteria cells, but their fragments. Various methods, including fermentation (in which case preparations are called ferment lysates), can be used to obtain such bacterial preparations. Bacterial cell fragments interact with the receptors of skin cells, enhancing local immunity and production of anti-inflammatory factors, and can also play the role of nutrients for other bacteria, i.e., prebiotics.

As for prebiotics *per se*, it has cost scientists a lot of effort to create a nutrition medium that stimulates the growth of saprophytic bacteria, but not pathogenic and opportunistic microflora. Typical prebiotics include inulin, fructooligosaccharides, galactooligosaccharides, and lactulose. These have gradually been supplemented with xylooligosaccharides, long chain β-glucans, and glucomannan.

Examples of synbiotics include these most frequently used combinations:

- Inulin + *Lactobacillus*
- Xylooligosaccharides + *Lactobacillus*, *Streptococcus*, and *Bifidobacterium*
- Lactosucrose + *Lactobacillus* and *Bifidobacterium*

The effectiveness of pre- and probiotics in treating skin pathologies has been actively studied, and the results obtained are impressive. For example, topical application of cream with *Lactobacillus plantarum* on acne-affected skin helps to reduce the number of inflammatory elements and erythema, and topical application of *Vitreoscilla filiformis* lysates reduces inflammation and significantly improves the course of atopic and seborrheic dermatitis compared to placebo (Muizzuddin N. et al., 2012; Mottin V.H.M., Syenaga E.S., 2018). A cream containing *Bifidobacterium longum* extract was found to decrease the reactivity of hypersensitive skin in an experiment conducted by Guéniche A., Bastien P., et al. (2010).

Reports show that glucooligosaccharides are capable of successfully controlling *Staphylococcus aureus* skin population in atopic dermatitis (Blanchet-Réthoré S. et al., 2017). Different formulations with β-glucans have been shown to improve wound healing, ameliorate skin dryness, and reduce itching in bacterial infections (Kiousi D.E. et al., 2019).

An essential factor in probiotic skincare products is the ability to maintain the pH level on the skin surface.

6.5. Special cosmetic ingredients for rosacea

Ingredients with anti-inflammatory and soothing properties can help reduce inflammation and calm the skin. Some plant extracts rich in polyphenols and antioxidants (chamomile, aloe, centella, and many others) have such properties and have traditionally been popular ingredients in cosmetics.

Among the new and promising developments in rosacea therapy are agents that inhibit the activity of TRPV receptors: peptides Skinasensyl® (INCI: Aqua (and) Glycerin (and) Coco-Glucoside (and) **Acetyl Tetrapeptide-15**) and Calmosensine® (Butylene Glycol (and) Aqua (and) Laureth-3 (and) Hydroxyethylcellulose (and) **Acetyl Dipeptide-1 Cetyl Ester**), and Northern truffle (*Albatrellus ovinus*) extract.

6.5.1. Antioxidants

Antioxidants are natural or synthetic substances that can slow down oxidation. Because the skin with rosacea has both a deficiency in its antioxidant defenses and an excess of ROS, using these compounds is very important.

An antioxidant can lower the number of ROS and prevent the development of radical chain reactions. Usually, an antioxidant sacrifices itself, i.e., reacts with ROS, transforming it into a chemically stable and inactive molecule. In doing so, the antioxidant becomes a free radical, but is chemically much less active (**Fig. I-6-5**). In this form, it is not dangerous to its surroundings, but it is also not functional until it is restored to its active state. Thus, the **antioxidant molecule, once reacted, loses its potency**.

In a reduction–oxidation (redox) reaction, an electron transfer occurs from the reducing agent (electron donor) to the oxidizing agent (electron acceptor)

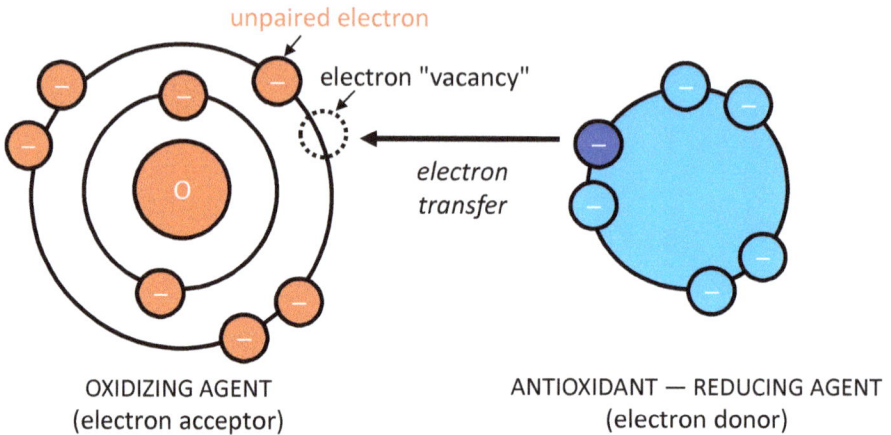

unpaired electron

electron "vacancy"

O

electron transfer

OXIDIZING AGENT
(electron acceptor)

ANTIOXIDANT — REDUCING AGENT
(electron donor)

Figure I-6-5. The antioxidant gives its electron to the free radical, thereby reducing it to a stable form

Our body synthesizes most antioxidants, and replenishes them as needed, but some of them (e.g., vitamin C, flavonoids, selenium) come from food. In the case of rosacea, the body's antioxidant system is weakened, so using external antioxidants is very important.

Antioxidants differ in their potency, "targets," and mechanisms of action. In addition, some are oil-soluble and "work" in the lipid phase (in membranes, they prevent lipid peroxidation). At the same time, another part is water-soluble and protects water-soluble compounds from free-radical attacks.

The greatest antioxidant effect is achieved when antioxidants act in pairs or groups. After giving up its electron to the free radical, the antioxidant is oxidized and rendered inactive. To return it to its working state, it must be restored. Thus, glutathione restores vitamin C, which in turn restores vitamin E.

Popular antioxidants:

- Vitamin C
- Vitamin E
- β-Carotene
- α-Lipoic acid (thioctic acid)

- Coenzyme Q_{10} (ubiquinone)
- *Maritime pine* bark extract
- Green tea extract
- *Euterpe oleracea* fruit (Acai berry) extract
- *Polypodium leucotomos* fern extract
- *Centella asiatica* extract
- Resveratrol

Many antioxidants also have anti-inflammatory and soothing properties.

6.5.2. Zinc

Zinc preparations dry the skin, reduce sebum production (by acting on 5α-reductase), and attenuate the inflammatory process. Zinc inhibits TLR receptors in the keratinocytes and dendritic cells (Langerhans cells) (Maywald M. et al., 2017). These receptors, directly involved in the rosacea pathogenesis, can be conceived of as the "levers" through which zinc can trigger various biochemical processes at the cellular level, ultimately reducing the severity of the inflammatory response in the skin tissue.

However, zinc salts' solubility is low, making it challenging to introduce them in formulations. Zinc pyroglutamate (zinc salt of pyroglutamic acid; also known as pyrrolidone carboxylic acid or PCA) is free from this disadvantage. PCA belongs to organic acids and plays an important role in the maturation of corneocytes and maintenance of the water balance in the *stratum corneum*. It is derived from the amino acid glutamine, which is released in large quantities during the hydrolysis of filaggrin as a part of keratinization. Subsequently, PCA is synthesized from glutamine via g-glutamyl-AA-synthase and g-glutamyl transferase. In the form of sodium or potassium salt, it is part of the natural moisturizing factor and facilitates water binding within the *stratum corneum*. Thus, zinc pyroglutamate also acts as a moisturizing agent, which is very important for oily skin. Zinc pyroglutamate (often paired with nicotinamide) can be found in many care cosmetics for oily skin (Gammoh N.Z., Rink L., 2017).

6.5.3. Niacinamide

Niacin (nicotinic acid) and niacinamide (nicotinamide) are two forms of vitamin B_3 (**Fig. I-6-6**). In the human body, niacin is converted to niacinamide. But this happens only when ingested, so both forms of vitamin B_3 can occur in vitamin supplements.

There is no transformation of niacin into amide when applied to the skin. Moreover, after topical application of these two forms, their impacts on the skin will differ. The main difference lies in the vasodilatory effect of niacin, which manifests in redness, whereas niacinamide does not cause such an effect.

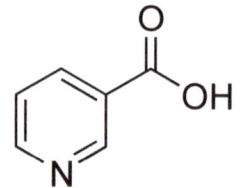

Niacin (nicotinic acid)

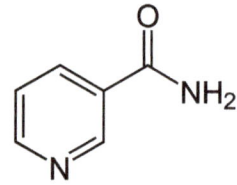

Niacinamide (nicotinamide)

Figure I-6-6. Forms of vitamin B_3

It should also be noted that, when taken orally, niacin in high doses can also lead to outbreaks of skin redness. Accordingly, vitamin supplements and topical agents containing niacin should be avoided in rosacea, even in the initial stages of the disease when the skin vessels are dilated due to impaired innervation of the vascular wall. Niacinamide, on the other hand, is safe in this regard and can provide many benefits.

Topical niacinamide stimulates the synthesis of ceramides, free fatty acids, and cholesterol, strengthening the lipid barrier. It improves energy metabolism in skin cells, normalizes metabolic processes, and exhibits antioxidant properties. All these factors positively affect the condition and appearance of the skin, as the tone is evened and inflammation subsides. In oily skin, there is a slight decrease in the sebum production activity. Preparations with niacinamide are also prescribed for injured skin, as niacinamide has a wound-healing effect (Draelos Z.D. et al., 2005; Wohlrab J., Kreft D., 2014; Chhabra G. et al., 2019). All these properties are advantageous in rosacea irrespective of the disease stage.

6.5.4. Tranexamic acid

Tranexamic acid (**Fig. I-6-7**) — a drug used to treat or prevent excessive blood loss from trauma, surgery, hemophilia, and heavy menstrual bleeding — is relatively new to aesthetic medicine. Still, it has already established itself as an effective treatment for rosacea and pigmentation.

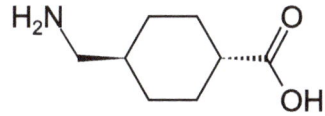

Figure I-6-7. Tranexamic acid

Such diversity of topical effects of tranexamic acid is associated with its unique mechanism of action: it blocks the plasminogen activator released by keratinocytes under the influence of UVB radiation. Yes, it is true: under UVB rays not only do endothelial cells release plasminogen activator at the rupture of the vessel wall (which is necessary for the formation of fibrin clot), but also keratinocytes! The epidermal plasminogen activator is responsible for excessive capillary growth in rosacea, pigmentation, and even inflammation (**Fig. I-6-8**).

In addition, a randomized placebo-controlled split-face study involving 30 patients with rosacea showed that tranexamic acid improves

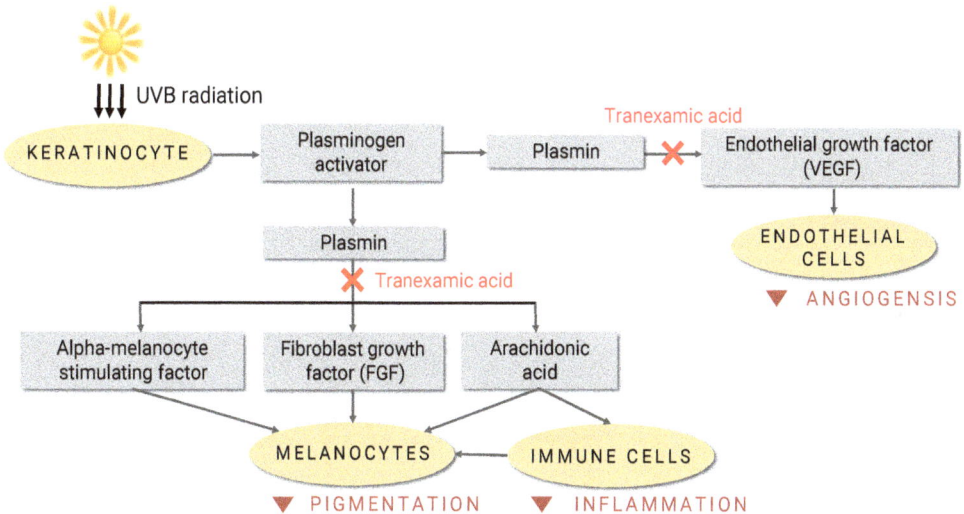

Figure I-6-8. Complex blockade of erythema, pigmentation, and inflammation by topical tranexamic acid

skin barrier function (Zhong S. et al., 2015). Study participants applied a 5% tranexamic acid solution to one side of the face twice daily for two weeks and a placebo solution to the other (control). The measured skin physiological parameters — such as skin surface pH, *stratum corneum* hydration, and transepidermal water loss — were significantly improved on the tranexamic acid-treated side.

Tranexamic acid is non-toxic and does not irritate hypersensitive skin (Forbat E. et al., 2020). It is claimed that tranexamic acid and niacinamide complement each other in caring for rosacea-affected skin.

6.5.5. Azelaic acid

Azelaic acid (**Fig. I-6-9**) is used not only as a medicinal ingredient but also as a cosmetic ingredient. The anti-inflammatory effects of azelaic acid are particularly useful

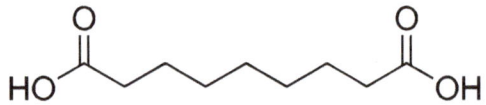

Figure I-6-9. Azelaic acid

in rosacea. It inhibits the production of major pro-inflammatory cytokines (IL-1 and -8, TGFα), which helps reduce skin reactivity in all stages of rosacea (Mastrofrancesco A. et al., 2010).

6.6. Sunscreen products

Using sunscreens is essential for rosacea management and maintenance of rosacea remission. In the previously mentioned US National Rosacea Society study, 81% of participants reported that sunlight triggered flare-ups, making the vascular pattern (telangiectasia) more pronounced and the erythema more vivid. Due to the proven link between exacerbations and sunlight, the general recommendation for all patients with rosacea is the use of sunscreen with sun protection factor (SPF) 15 or higher when exposed to the sun at any time of year (in summer, the SPF should be at least 30, and preferably 50).

1. **Protection against UVA/B radiation.** UV filters can be classified into two groups according to their nature. The inorganic UV filters (also called physical UV filters) principally work by reflecting and

scattering the UV radiation, while the organic UV filters (also called chemical UV filters) absorb the light. Physical UV filters' irritating potential is lower compared to the chemical ones'. Chemical UV filters such as benzophenone-3 (aka oxybenzone), benzophenone-4, avobenzone, octocrylene, and para-aminobenzoic acid (PABA) are potentially irritant (Diffey B., 2020).

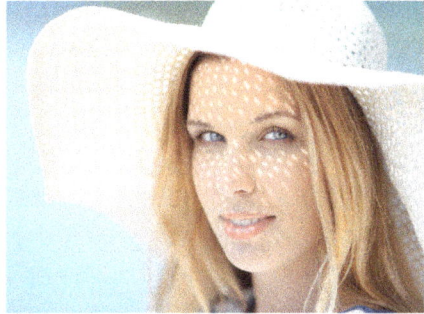

2. Experts recommend **using sunscreen daily**, regardless of whether the sun is shining or the weather is overcast. This is the only way to ensure the skin is not exposed to excessive UV "load." We still recommend being guided by the UV index*: if it is higher than 3, the sunscreen should be used.

3. The **best sun protection** is nonetheless achieved with clothing, hat, and shade.

Sunscreen formulations include substances that impart additional properties to the finished product. These include moisturizing components, anti-inflammatory agents, antioxidants (usually oil-soluble vitamin E), and immunomodulators (yeast polysaccharides, chitosan). The main thing here is not to overdo it. There is a general rule: the higher the degree of photoprotection, the fewer additional "active" substances in the formulation there should be. There is an explanation for this advice: a sunscreen product that provides high photoprotection for a long time should restrain the "pressure" of ultraviolet light, which means that everything that can potentially increase skin photosensitivity should be avoided. Fragrances and dyes are also highly undesirable.

Another nuance is the introduction of anti-inflammatory agents in sunscreens. Since the only sign of pronounced photodamage to

---

* The **ultraviolet index**, or **UV index**, is an international standard measurement of the strength of the sunburn-producing ultraviolet (UV) radiation at a particular place and time. It is primarily used in daily and hourly forecasts for the public (Wikipedia).

the skin is erythema, and they "take it away," there are concerns that their presence in the formula may give people a sense of false security. People may mistakenly assume that "Since my skin isn't red yet, it means the sunscreen is working, and I'm protected," when that may not be true.

However, the photostable antioxidants in the formula are welcome. They not only do not reduce the sun protection capacity of the product, but also strengthen the skin's defense against UV-induced free radicals. Vitamin E protects skin cells from forming "dark" cyclobutene pyrimidine dimers and oxidatively generated DNA damage (Delinasios G.J. et al., 2018).

Some sunscreens formulated for rosacea-affected skin are multifunctional and can act as both moisturizers and concealers. Their moisturizing properties are mostly related to emollients, whereas masking is achieved by color pigments, mainly green pigments, which "neutralize" the red color. So, they can be used as a base for makeup as well.

Ideally, it is best to avoid sun exposure between 10 am and 4 pm, when the sun is at its peak. The product should be reapplied after swimming or sweating. Remember that UV exposure increases in the presence of reflective surfaces (snow, water, white sand) and that, as said before, the best sunscreen is clothing, hat, and shade.

It is also important to note that some commonly used medications can increase skin photosensitivity. We have listed the most common photosensitizers that can cause phototoxic (associated with direct cellular damage and accelerating sunburn) and photoallergic (dermatitis-like immune reaction) reactions in **Table I-6-1**. It is essential to inquire about the use of these products (and even perfume use) during the patient's history collection. In all these situations, products with the highest protection factor should be recommended, and it is best if they use physical UV filters such as titanium dioxide and zinc oxide.

Table I-6-1. Photosensitizing drugs

GROUP	DRUGS	PHOTOTOXIC REACTION	PHOTOALLERGIC REACTION
Antibiotics	Tetracyclines (doxycy-cline, tetracycline)	Yes	No
	Fluoroquinolones (ciprofloxacin, ofloxacin, levofloxacin)	Yes	No
	Sulfonamides	Yes	No
Antivirals	Acyclovir	No	Yes
Non-steroidal anti-inflam-matory drugs	Ibuprofen	Yes	No
	Ketoprofen	Yes	Yes
	Naproxen	Yes	No
	Celecoxib	No	Yes
Hormonal drugs	Hydrocortisone	No	Yes
Diuretics	Furosemide	Yes	No
	Bumetanide	No	No
	Hydrochlorthiazide	Yes	No
Retinoids	Isotretinoin	Yes	No
	Acitretin	Yes	No
Hypoglycemic drugs	Sulfonylureas (glipizide, glyburide)	No	Yes
HMG-CoA reductase inhibitors	Statins (atorvastatin, fluvastatin, lovastatin, pravastatin, simvastatin)	Yes	Yes
EGF inhibitors	Cetuximab, panitumum-ab, erlotinib, gefitinib, lapatinib,vandetanib	Yes	Yes
Antifungals	Terbinafine	No	No
	Itraconazole	Yes	Yes
	Voriconazole	Yes	No
	Griseofulvin	Yes	Yes

Continued on p. 82

GROUP	DRUGS	PHOTOTOXIC REACTION	PHOTOALLERGIC REACTION
Antipsychotic drugs	Phenothiazines (chlor-promazine, fluphen-azine, fluphenazine, perazine, perphen-azine, thioridazine)	Yes	Yes
	Thioxanthenes (chlorprothixene, thiothixene)	Yes	No
Different drugs	5-Fluorouracil	Yes	Yes
	Paclitaxel	Yes	No
	Amiodarone	Yes	No
	Diltiazem	Yes	No
	Quinidine	Yes	Yes
	Hydroxychloroquine	No	No
	Nifedipine	Yes	No
	Enalapril	No	No
	Dapson	No	Yes
	Oral contraceptives	No	Yes
Alpha-hy-droxy acids	Glycolic acid	Yes (in high concentration)	Yes
Sunscreens	Para-aminobenzoic acid	No	Yes
	Cinnamic acid esters (cinnamates)	No	Yes
	Benzophenones	No	Yes
	Salicylates	No	Yes
Flavorings	Amber musk (ambre-tol)	No	Yes
	6-methylcoumarin	No	Yes
	Essential oils (berga-mot, cumin, ginger, lemon, lime, tangerine, orange, and verbena)	No (bergamot yes)	Yes

6.7. Decorative cosmetics

While therapeutic measures affect physiological processes deep within the skin, makeup simply improves its appearance which in turn has a positive effect on the patient's psychological condition. It can be said that makeup is an element of psychotherapy, and its use on sensitive skin with rosacea significantly improves the life quality of patients.

Here are a few simple rules for the effective use of decorative cosmetics to mask rosacea symptoms.

1. **Prepare your skin before applying makeup.** The skin should be cleaned and moisturized.
2. **Makeup application.** Tonal cream (foundation) should be applied with fingertips only, without rubbing or stretching the skin. Brushes for applying dry products (blush, powder, shadow) should be soft and preferably have an antibacterial coating.
3. **Choosing a foundation.** Foundation should have a greenish tint as green pigments "neutralize" the red color and visually even out the skin tone. Modern foundations can contain physical UV filters, which is an additional argument for choosing a product. The presence of organic oils in the composition of the foundation is undesirable. First, they can oxidize and provoke lipid peroxidation in the skin in sunlight. Second, they are sticky, which worsens the subsequent application of loose powder.

6.7.1. How to apply makeup to minimize irritation

- **Foundation.** Apply foundation with light strokes, taking care not to rub the skin. You can use a brush with an antibacterial coating. Still, it is necessary to remember that after use, it must be washed to keep it clean until the next time.
- **Concealer and corrector*.** These products are applied before the foundation using a thin brush with an antibacterial coating.

---

* Corrector helps to cover dark areas like black spots or dark circles. Concealer helps merge and hide the corrector that has been used. In cases where a corrector is not used, it covers dullness and lights darkness / redness on the face.

- **Camouflage cosmetics.** In moderate and severe forms of rosacea, and when redness is pronounced, camouflage cosmetics will help reduce the disease's visual signs.
- **Mineral powder.** It is recommended to apply yellowish mineral powder on top of your foundation. It reduces oily shine and gives your skin a healthier tone. In addition, physical UVA/B filters are found in mineral powders.
- **Blush.** Dry mineral-based blushes are commercially available and are safe for the rosacea-affected skin. However, blush can only emphasize the redness. If you decide to use blush, apply it with an antibacterial brush.
- **Eye makeup.** Choose products that have undergone special ophthalmologic testing. Mascara should be easily washed off with water. Mineral shadows are suitable for people even with ocular rosacea. Shadows and pencils of neutral colors can be less irritating than bright products, because they have less pigment.
- **Lipstick.** Avoid lipstick in bright red shades, as it will further emphasize the redness of the face. Give preference to neutral light colors.

Chapter 7
Energy-based methods

Most current physical treatments for rosacea focus on destroying growing blood capillaries. Apart from the obvious advantage of this approach in eliminating the key "target" of this pathology, the effects of physical treatment are usually seen within a limited number of sessions, which contrasts with the need for prolonged daily administration of topical or oral products. Once the desired therapeutic effects have been achieved, the results usually persist for several years. Still, given that any damage is associated with regenerative processes, including angiogenesis, the process of new vessel formation continues, and the disease may return.

The primary physiotherapeutic method for treating rosacea is light therapy using lasers and intense pulsed light (IPL) devices as discussed in detail below.

7.1. Light therapy: mechanism of action

The ability of light to affect specific skin targets was noted in the earliest studies of the laser effect on human skin. However, the transformation of these observations into applied technologies became possible with the greater understanding of the scientific principles behind these effects. In this context, the **selective photothermolysis** theory put forward by Richard Rox Anderson and John Parrish of the Wellman Center for Photomedicine at Harvard Medical School (Anderson R.R., Parrish J.A., 1983) was particularly impactful.

Their idea was to apply a laser beam to a chromophore substance that absorbs certain types of electromagnetic radiation better than others and the concentration of which in the target cell is much higher

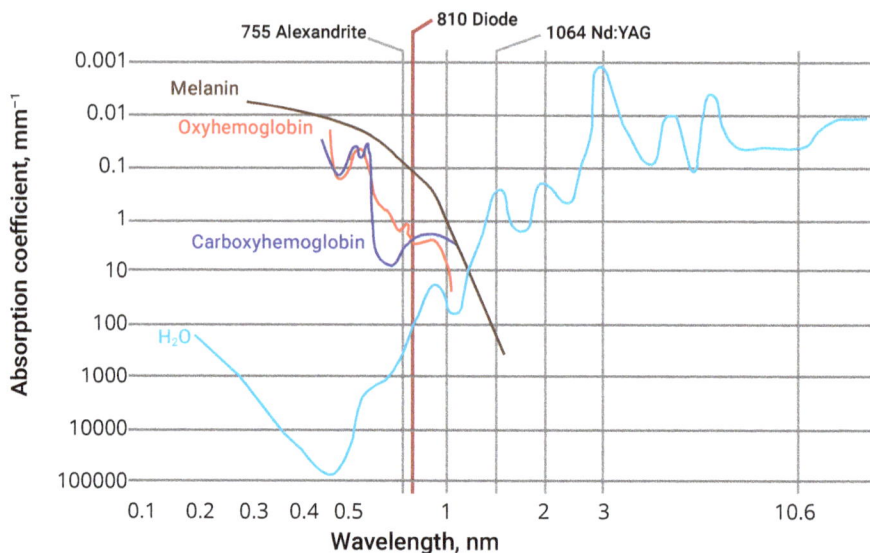

Figure I-7-1. Absorption spectra of skin chromophores

than in neighboring cells (**Fig. I-7-1**). The light parameters (wavelength, intensity, and duration of exposure) are tailored to the absorption spectrum of the chromophore to transfer as much energy as possible to its molecules. After absorbing light, the chromophore enters an excited state, whereas the reverse transition is accompanied by the dissipation of excess energy to the surrounding space in the form of heat. Thus, under incident light, heating occurs, causing irreversible destruction of both the target and the cell in which it is located and, if necessary, its immediate neighbors (**enhanced selective photothermolysis**).

In rosacea, the target chromophore is blood erythrocyte hemoglobin (for destruction of vascular structures) or water (for phymatous tissue destruction and remodeling).

In the first case, special selective vascular lasers are used. By absorbing their radiation, hemoglobin is heated, and the vessel walls are also heated, which leads to their coagulation (photothermal effect) or rupture (photomechanical effect).

- **The photomechanical effect** occurs when a large amount of energy is transferred to the chromophore quickly. The resulting so-called photodynamic shock causes the vessel to rupture and release its contents into tissues, leading to the formation of purpura, petechiae, and bruises.

■ **The photothermal effect** is induced with slower heating of the target (longer pulse) with gradual adhesion (coagulation) of the vessel. Blood, subjected to photocoagulation, forms a thermal coagulum — an amorphous accumulation of damaged and agglutinated erythrocytes and plasma components that clog the vascular lumen. Histologically, selective vessel damage with thrombosis, necrosis of the vessel walls, and perivascular collagen damage with relatively minor thermal damage to the epidermis and dermis is noted. The final step will be thrombosis and vessel occlusion (Weinkle A.P. et al., 2015).

Besides vascular lasers targeting hemoglobin, non-selective lasers are used to treat rosacea. In this case, the chromophore will be water, but because water is present in all cells, the effect will not be restricted to some individual targets.

Non-selective photothermolysis is based on **photoablation**, i.e., almost instantaneous tissue evaporation at high temperatures, or **photocoagulation** at less pronounced heating. For ablation to occur, the tissue must be rapidly heated to several hundred degrees Celsius.

Fig. I-7-2 shows a plot of light absorption by tissues and water as a function of radiation wavelength. It is easy to see that the tissues' absorption spectrum correlates with the water's absorption spectrum. Radiation from the far-infrared (IR) and ultraviolet (UV) regions of the spectrum is best absorbed by the body tissues, which means that its penetration beyond the surface layer will be minimal, and all light energy will be released as heat in a minimal volume of tissue. For obvious reasons,

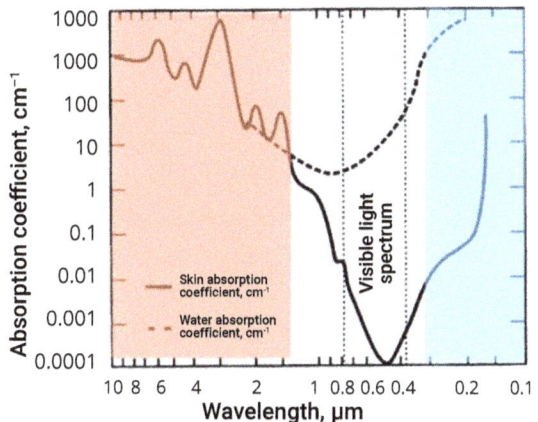

Figure I-7-2. Absorption spectra of the skin and water

UV light cannot be used for heating, because it is harmful in high doses. However, far-IR radiation has no such contraindications, so this part of the spectrum is used in ablative treatment. Such procedures rely on carbon dioxide (CO_2), erbium:yttrium-aluminum-garnet crystal (Er:YAG), and erbium:yttrium-scandium-gallium-garnet crystal (Er:YSGG) lasers, which are appropriately named **ablative** and involve damage to the *stratum corneum*. Water molecules also absorb near-IR radiation, though less actively; this is the radiation of Diode (1440 nm), neodymium:yttrium-aluminum-garnet crystal (Nd:YAG; 1320, 1440 nm), fiber Er:glass (1540 and 1550 nm) and Thulium (1927 nm) lasers. As their energy is not high enough for ablation, they work through coagulation without damaging the *stratum corneum* and are classified as **non-ablative**.

In addition to single-wavelength (monochrome) lasers, IPL devices are also used to destroy vascular defects of rosacea. IPL devices emit a wide range of wavelengths that various skin chromophores absorb. Still, surface targets such as melanin spots and dilated vessels absorb most of this energy. IPL therapy can be beneficial in treating rosacea, especially in the initial stage of the disease.

7.2. Laser and IPL devices

Depending on the clinical manifestations of rosacea, two light therapy approaches can be distinguished (**Table I-7-1**):
1) treating vascular and inflammatory skin problems
2) treating tissue dystrophic changes

There are several factors to consider to increase the chances of obtaining the most optimal results:
- **Vessel diameter:** as a rule, vessels 0.1–3 mm in diameter are most effectively treated.
- **Vessel depth:** the superficial vasculature is affected by short-wave radiation (532, 577, and 585 nm), and vessels below the reticular dermis are affected by long-wave radiation (600, 755, 800, and 1064 nm).
- **Skin phototype and pigmentation in the exposed area:** melanin is an oxyhemoglobin-competing chromophore. When

Table I-7-1. Lasers for rosacea treatment

TARGET PROCESS	DEVICE	EXPECTED RESULT
Vascular changes	• Pulsed dye laser (PDL, 585–595 nm) • Intense pulsed light (IPL, 500–1200 nm) • Potassium-titanium-phosphate laser (KTP, 532, 540 nm) • Neodymium laser (Nd:YAG, 1064 nm)	Reduction in the severity of clinical symptoms, removal of telangiectasias and erythema
Inflammation	• PDL (585–595 nm) • KTP (532, 540 nm)	Reduction in rashes, rapid achievement, and maintenance of remission
Deformational, hypertrophic changes	• Carbon dioxide laser (CO_2, 10,600 nm) • Er:YAG laser (2900 nm) • Nd:YAG laser (1064 nm)	Correction of the shape of altered anatomical formations
Dystrophic changes	**Ablative fractional lasers** • CO_2 laser (10,600 nm) • Er:YAG laser (2940 nm) **Non-ablative fractional lasers** • Diode and Neodymium lasers (1440 nm) • Thulium laser (1927 nm) • Erbium laser (1550 nm)	Reduction in the severity of clinical symptoms, achievement of long-term remission

treating skin with high melanin levels, it is necessary to use skin cooling during light therapy.

■ **Size of the light spot:** the larger the size of the light spot, the deeper the radiation penetration into the tissue. The small-spot-size radiation has less penetrating ability but necessitates the use of more energy for the entire vascular removal procedure.

■ **Energy flux density:** the density of light radiation per unit area needs to be considered. While it is important to use a high energy flux density, the optimal value should be determined by the vessel's color change (as a rule, it darkens).

■ **Pulse duration:** for effective and safe impact on the vessel, the pulse should be less than or equal to the duration of the vessel's thermal relaxation time (TRT), as a pulse exceeding the TRT of the vessel causes the spread of heat to the surrounding tissue, which can lead to its coagulation.

- **Limiting insolation before and after the light therapy** is required to avoid the formation of pigment spots.

7.3. Treating vascular alterations

- Pulsed dye laser (PDL; 585–595 nm)
- Potassium-titanium-phosphate laser (KTP; 532, 540 nm)
- Neodymium laser (Nd:YAG; 1064 nm)
- Intense pulsed light (IPL; 500–1200 nm)

Pulsed dye laser (PDL)

Pulsed dye laser is considered the "gold standard" for treating vascular skin disorders. PDL wavelengths (577, 585, 595 nm) coincide with the absorption peak of hemoglobin and thus affect the superficial vascular network, making them very effective in destroying superficial vascular defects, although not effective enough to remove deep-seated vessels.

Studies show a favorable effect of this type of radiation in erythema and telangiectasia, as well as in rash reduction in the papulopustular rosacea. An anti-inflammatory effect has also been noted. Immuno-histochemical investigations performed by Seaton E.D. and colleagues in 2006 further indicate that a statistically significant decrease in neuropeptides involved in the microvascular pathophysiological reaction can be sustained up to three months after the laser session, contributing to the anti-inflammatory effects.

Previously, the main disadvantage of classical PDL lasers was the occurrence of purpura and dyschromia after treatment, which has now been minimized by increasing the pulse duration (Weinkle A.P. et al., 2015).

Potassium-titanium-phosphate laser (KTP)

KTP (operating at 532 and 540 nm wavelengths) is ideal for removing linear and branching telangiectasias at various depths. Green light is in the absorption spectrum of hemoglobin, which allows a significant part of the energy to be directed to the coagulation of vessels of different diameters.

Available evidence indicates that KTP is effective in treating facial erythema, telangiectasias, and papulopustular rash, while also decreasing the severity of the inflammatory response. Subjective sensations such as soreness, purpura, and hyperpigmentation after KTP therapy are insignificant and usually transient.

The disadvantage is that radiation at these wavelengths is absorbed not just by hemoglobin but also by melanin, which increases the risk of pigmentation disorders (Weinkle A.P. et al., 2015).

Fig. I-7-3 shows clinical cases.

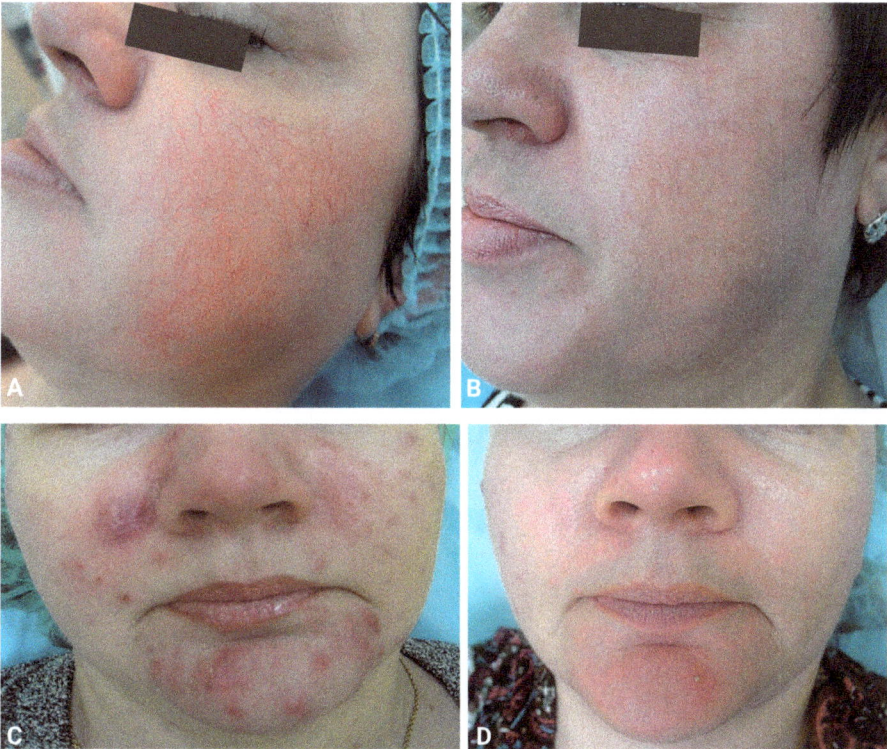

Figure I-7-3. Top: Erythematotelangiectatic rosacea: (A) before treatment and (B) three months after five sessions of laser vascular coagulation (Nd:YAP/KTP/Q-switched, 540 nm) two weeks apart. Bottom: Rosacea papulopustulosa: (C) before treatment and (D) three months after five sessions of laser treatment (Nd:YAP/KTP/Q-switched, 540 nm) two weeks apart (Photo: Kalashnikova N.G., Urakova D.S.)

Neodymium laser (Nd:YAG)

Nd:YAG (1064 nm) allows the treatment of large and deep vessels, which is typically required to remove blood vessels in the legs. It is also the device of choice when working with dark skin phototypes. The disadvantages are the transient presence of purpura and soreness, and occasional burns due to tissue "overheating" (Say E.M. et al., 2015; Weinkle A.P. et al., 2015; Seo H.-M. et al., 2016).

Intense pulsed light (IPL)

IPL devices (operating at 500–1200 nm wavelengths) are applicable in various clinical situations. Their use allows the removal of both superficial and deep-lying vessels (at specific exposure parameters), which leads to a reduction in the severity of erythema and telangiectasia. Still, IPL application requires the specialist's clinical knowledge and practical experience to properly select the settings for the procedure and reduce the risk of complications. The likelihood of complications when using high-energy treatment settings increases due to the active exposure to many chromophores in the skin (melanin, hemoglobin, protein, water) (Weinkle A.P. et al., 2015). Studies conducted with patients in the early stages of rosacea confirm a positive effect in 75–100% of cases after one or two sessions, with few complications in the form of purpura, scarring, and post-inflammatory hyperpigmentation (Weinkle A.P. et al., 2015).

7.4. Treating connective tissue changes

7.4.1. Dissection of altered anatomical entities

Rhinophyma is a severe late complication of rosacea characterized by progressive hyperplasia of sebaceous glands and connective tissue with involvement of the lower two-thirds of the nose (Kassir R. et al., 2012).

Rosacea treatment is usually conservative and can only manage the course of the disease. Currently available drugs can reduce the severity of erythematoteleangiectatic, papulopustular, and ocular manifestations, but there is no convincing evidence that drugs can cause regression of rhinophyma. In this case, invasive techniques remain the best choice for treating deformed tissue (Campolmi P. et al., 2012; Kassir R. et al., 2012; Weinkle A.P. et al., 2015).

Laser resurfacing, a dissection of deformed tissue with a continuous laser beam, can be performed with the following types of lasers emitting in the IR spectal region:
- Carbon dioxide laser (CO_2; 10,600 nm)
- Erbium laser (Er:YAG; 2900 nm)
- Neodymium laser (Nd:YAG; 1064 nm)

IR radiation is well absorbed by water and causes heating. In addition IR-emitting lasers provide a precise, effective, and targeted thermal effect on the lesions, thus guaranteeing optimal re-epithelialization. This makes them suitable for surgical interventions with a limited inflammatory response as their use promotes tissue healing (Campolmi P. et al., 2012; Kassir R. et al., 2012).

CO_2 laser, unlike Erbium laser, induces the most traumatic changes in tissues, but can provide a dry wound surface during surgery. As for the Neodymium emitter, it is also able to provide complete coagulation of vessels and "dry" surgical field, which undoubtedly contributes to a favorable aesthetic effect, but its cutting properties are lower than those of CO_2 laser (Urakova D.S., Fominykh E.M., 2011; Kalashnikova N.G., 2014).

Ablative laser therapy can be used to equalize the shape of a deformed nose by partial excision of excess tissue. Despite transient edema, erythema, crusting, and the risk of pigmentation disorders and scarring, the results can be aesthetically and psychologically acceptable (Campolmi P. et al., 2012; Kassir R. et al., 2012).

Rhinophyma causes significant psychological and physiological problems for patients, but there is no ideal solution for its removal. Some scientists and practitioners advocate for a combined therapy in the form of surgical cytoreduction and fractional photothermolysis, which minimizes the risks of complications and gives better short- and long-term results (Campolmi P. et al., 2012; Kassir R. et al., 2012; Weinkle A.P. et al., 2015).

7.4.2. Tissue remodeling

Ablative and non-ablative fractional lasers are used to remodel the altered tissue.

Ablative fractional lasers
- Carbon dioxide (CO_2) laser (10,600 nm)
- Er:YAG laser (2940 nm)
- Er:YAG laser with the spatially modulated ablation (SMA) module (2940 nm)

Lasers in this group operate in the mid- and far-IR range, with water serving as the primary chromophore. The principle of fractional treatment is based on the formation of multiple microchannels in the skin through thermal damage, with the treated areas surrounded by intact skin. The microchannels pass through the epidermis and reach the dermis. Damage to the skin triggers healing and renewal processes. As a result of intensive exfoliation of the epidermis, the skin becomes lighter and more even, as the remodeling of the dermal matrix makes the skin tighter and shrinks enlarged pores (Kassir R. et al., 2012; Kalashnikova N.G., 2014).

Erbium laser with SMA module exerts an effect with a leading photomechanical mechanism. Acoustic waves propagate into the dermal layer of the skin, causing interferential micro-traumatization of cell membranes and unfolding of connective tissue fibers. In response, reparative processes are activated with connective tissue remodeling (Kalashnikova N.G., 2014; Urakova D.S., Kalashnikova N.G., 2015; Seo H.-M. et al., 2016). a clinical case is presented in **Fig. I-7-4**.

In contrast to classical ablative lasers, recovery following fraction treatment is faster, and the inflammatory process is not as pronounced, which reduces the risk of scarring and dyschromia.

Non-ablative fractional lasers
- Diode and Neodymium lasers (1440 nm)
- Thulium laser (1927 nm)
- Erbium laser (1550 nm)

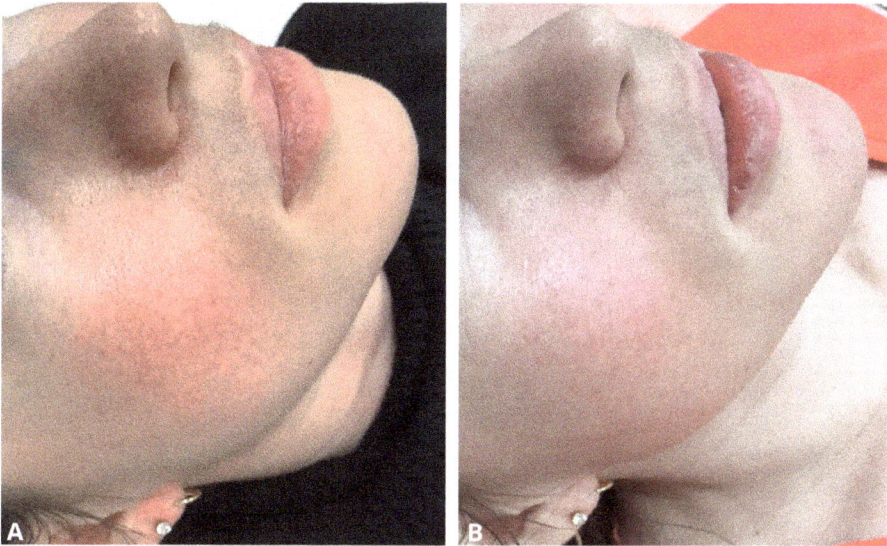

Figure I-7-4. Erythematotelangiectatic rosacea: (A) before treatment and (B) two months after a single session (Er:YAG with SMA-module 2940 nm) (Photo: Kalashnikova N.G., Urakova D.S.)

These lasers target water-containing tissue, creating coagulation zones in the dermis. The *stratum corneum* remains intact during the session, and no visible wound surface is formed. After exposure, erythema and edema appear on the skin, accompanied by soreness, but these phenomena are usually short-lived. a remodeling effect accompanies recovery, but the risks of erythema, dyschromia, and scars are also present (Rakhanskaya E.M., 2016).

It should be noted that laser therapy for skin remodeling can be carried out only when the inflammatory response activity is completely reduced. The altered tissue structures are very sensitive to various stimuli and any existing changes may be exacerbated.

To maximize the satisfaction of rosacea patients, a combined approach consisting of sequentially addressing different objectives with medication and light therapy is preferable (Campolmi P. et al., 2012; Kassir R. et al., 2012).

7.5. RF microneedling

There have been reports on the effectiveness of fractional radio-frequency (RF) microneedling in treating rosacea (Ahn T.H., Cho S.B., 2017). RF heating is currently one of the most popular techniques, and is based on heating tissues by alternating electric currents of high frequency. During RF microneedling, the electric current is conducted into the skin through sharp needle electrodes. These needle electrodes are positively charged, and the lateral flat electrodes are negatively charged. Depending on the treated area's size and the wrinkles' depth, applicators with different needle densities are selected. When RF energy is applied to the needle electrodes, ablation (local removal of tissue with the formation of a crater) occurs. a coagulation zone forms around the crater, while cells are stimulated in the heating zone. After the formation of localized zones of damage in the skin, the process of regeneration and remodeling is initiated.

Park S.Y. et al. (2016) examined the mechanisms of RF microneedling in rosacea, noting that the positive effects of this method are associated with a reduction in inflammation and inhibition of angiogenesis. In their study, RF treatment reduced the expression of nuclear factor kappa light chain enhancer of activated B cells (NF-kB), IL-8, and VEGF. The procedures were also found to affect the immune and neurogenic component of the disease, namely decreased expression of TLR2, LL-37, and TRPV, as well as a detrimental effect on *Demodex* (Park S.Y. et al., 2016). However, as RF microneedling is an invasive procedure, it can provoke rosacea exacerbation in some cases (Aşiran Serdar Z., Aktaş Karabay E., 2019).

Chapter 8
Botulinum toxin therapy

Mesotherapy is not prescribed to treat rosacea, as it may cause skin damage. However, injectable botulinum toxin can be used for rosacea management, given that this drug has been actively studied as a potential therapeutic tool, with promising results.

Botulinum toxin is a neurotoxin produced by the anaerobic gram-positive spore-forming microorganism *Clostridium botulinum*. It blocks the release of acetylcholine, a mediator transmitting nerve impulses to the muscle cells. In the absence of a signal to contract, the muscle relaxes.

Botulinum therapy — which consists of injecting botulinum toxin into the target muscle — has been successfully used in the treatment of various conditions and diseases with a neuromuscular link in their pathogenesis. However, in addition to nerve endings, acetylcholine is also released from other biologically active substances, such as substance P, histamine, and CGRP. These substances affect blood vessel walls and trigger the neurogenic inflammation in the pathogenesis of chronic dermatoses, including acne and rosacea. In the skin, botulinum toxin has been shown to inhibit the release of these substances from free nerve endings. This mechanism of action explains the therapeutic effect of intradermal micro-dose botulinum toxin injections in chronic inflammation and persistent erythema.

8.1. Mechanism of action

While the complex mechanisms underlying the clinical effects of botulinum toxin on rosacea are still unknown, it is suggested that inhibition of the release of acetylcholine and inflammatory mediators may be involved in modulating vascular dilatation and blood vessel wall permeability (Bansal C., et al., 2006; Carmichael N.M. et al., 2010).

Another possible mechanism concerns the effect of botulinum toxin on mast cells which, as we have already mentioned, are also actively involved in neurogenic inflammation in rosacea. The histamine released during their degranulation increases the permeability of the vascular wall and contributes to unpleasant sensations such as itching. Choi J.E. et al. (2019) studied the effect of botulinum toxin on human and mouse mast cells, and their findings indicate that pretreatment of these cells with botulinum toxin type a or B significantly inhibits degranulation.

As a part of their study, these scientists also induced a rosacea-like condition in mice using LL-37, which is secreted in excess in rosacea. Mice pre-treated with intradermal injection of onabotulinum toxin type a showed significantly less erythema. They also had less pronounced mast cell degranulation as well as decreased messenger ribonucleic acid (mRNA) expression of rosacea biomarkers such as KLK5, MMP9, and TRPV2, typically elevated in the disease (Choi J.E. et al., 2019).

These data suggest that onabotulotoxin type a reduces rosacea-related skin inflammation by directly inhibiting mast cell degranulation. Therefore, the authors concluded that intradermal administration of the botulinum toxin may help patients with refractory forms of rosacea. However, full-fledged clinical trials are needed to substantiate their findings and implement this approach in widespread practice.

8.2. Clinical experience

The efficacy of botulinum toxin therapy in rosacea is difficult to determine, given that there are very few reliable clinical studies focusing specifically on this issue. Indeed, as a part of their literature review published by an international expert panel, Scala J. et al. (2019) searched PubMed International Database of Medical and Biological Research with the aim of retrieving and analyzing all articles on the use of botulinum toxin for rosacea and facial hyperemia that had been published by April 2017. The authors found 39 such articles, the first of which dated to 2005, but only 30 papers met the criteria for inclusion in the final analysis.

The reviewed studies differed in the botulinum toxin dose applied during treatment, ranging from 1 to 6 IU per 1 cm^2 of the affected skin, number of sessions provided (one to three), and the interval between them, but in all cases positive results were reported.

Only one of the included articles pertained to a randomized controlled trial aimed at assessing the effects of botulinum neuroprotein (Odo M.E. et al., 2011). The study sample comprised 60 menopausal women experiencing menopausal hot flashes, 30 of whom were injected with botulinum toxin at a dose of 6.2 IU (0.04 mL) at each selected point of the skin. For the remaining 30 participants who served as the control group, saline solution was used at the same volume of 0.04 mL per injection point. At the follow-up performed 60 days after therapy completion, the patients that were included in the intervention group noted a significant decrease in the frequency and intensity of redness and sweating. Although sweating returned after 180 days, it was less intense than before the therapy.

The study conducted by Bloom B.S. et al. (2015) specifically focused on rosacea, and 15 participants were given a single injection of 15–45 IU botulinum toxin administered into the facial skin. The authors noted a statistically significant reduction in erythema compared to baseline at one, two, and three months after treatment ($p < 0.05$, $p < 0.001$, and $p < 0.05$, respectively).

A more recent search of the PubMed database revealed several articles that were published since April 2017 which was a cut-off date for the aforementioned review. It is encouraging to note that a number of double-blind, randomized trials (albeit with small patient cohorts) have been conducted in recent years. In one case, researchers studied the efficacy of botulinum toxin type a in nine patients with erythematotelangiectatic and papulopustular rosacea. Four participants received 20 IU botulinum toxin injections into the cheek skin, and the remaining five received saline solution. Four weeks after the treatment, the experimental group showed a significant reduction in rosacea symptoms compared to the baseline and the control group (Dayan S.H. et al., 2017).

Bharti J. et al. (2023) also assessed the effectiveness of botulinum toxin intradermal micro-dose injections (0.05 mL [10 IU in 1 mL] per 0.5 cm² of skin). Two weeks after the procedure, the researchers recorded a significant reduction in erythema, edema, redness flare-ups, and rash severity, along with noticeable pore shrinkage. These effects persisted for 3–4 months (Bharti J. et al., 2023).

A reduction in redness and improvement in subjective sensations was observed by Friedman O. et al. (2019) after the topical application of 100 IU of botulinum toxin a to the participants' facial skin pre-treated with a thermomechanical system that forms holes in the superficial layers of the skin.

While these findings are certainly beneficial, large-scale randomized controlled trials are necessary to provide further evidence on the clinical efficacy of botulinum toxin in treating rosacea. However, the currently known mechanisms of action suggest the positive effects of botulinum toxin. After all, it affects one of the critical links in the pathogenesis of the disease. Therefore, botulinum toxin therapy may be considered as a component of rosacea management, but additional research is needed to develop standard protocols.

8.3. Rosacea-like steroid dermatitis

Skin lightening is one of the desired clinical effects of topical steroids and the reason for their abuse by some individuals. Unfortunately, uncontrolled long-term use of these highly effective drugs leads to adverse events and complications such as skin atrophy, acneiform rashes, and persistent erythema. Yet, as cessation of steroid use worsens the skin condition, withdrawal is usually short-term. Botulinum therapy may help break this vicious cycle. In their paper published in the *Indian Dermatology Online Journal*, Katoch S. et al. (2022) described a clinical case of topical corticosteroid rosacea-like dermatitis that responded well to botulinum therapy and ended in complete clinical recovery.

Their case study involved a 39-year-old female patient who complained of facial skin rashes, redness and burning, and itching and irritation when exposed to sunlight. Her medical history included prolonged use of over-the-counter steroid creams for the treatment of pigment spots on the face. As discontinuation of the cream worsened the condition, the patient continued to use it intermittently for symptomatic relief. Clinical examination revealed papular rash and erythematous brown macules on her forehead and cheeks. There was diffuse erythema on the forehead, cheeks, and perioral area. Several telangiectasias were also visible and the cheeks, nose, and chin were covered with pigmented spots. Based on these findings, diagnosis of melasma, rosacea-like dermatitis was made. Accordingly, the prescribed therapy included oral doxycycline, oral antihistamines, topical pimecrolimus, hypoallergenic moisturizer, and sunscreen with physical UV filters. After six weeks, the patient reported overall symptom improvement and the disappearance of papular rash. However, she still had facial redness, melasma, and post-inflammatory hyperpigmentation.

For general facial rejuvenation, the patient also requested botulinum therapy. After the consultation, botulinum toxin micro-dose intradermal injections were administered on the entire face. Two weeks after the session, the patient reported a marked reduction in facial erythema and improved facial condition. Topical kojic acid and oral antioxidants were added to the therapy regimen, and topical pimecrolimus was reduced to three times per week. After six months, the patient reported a complete disappearance of erythema and improvement of melasma.

This clinical case is consistent with other observations of botulinum toxin therapy's efficacy in treating chronic inflammation and persistent erythema of neurogenic origin. As mentioned previously, botulinum toxin blocks the release of acetylcholine from peripheral autonomic nerves of the cutaneous vasculature, thereby modulating vasodilatory responses. It also inhibits mast cell degranulation and release of neuropeptides, substance P, and CGRP. This mechanism of action suppresses the influx of inflammatory mediators and gives the skin time to heal. Most importantly, the attained improvements are usually long-lasting, with no recurrence of symptoms.

In the presented case report, the patient responded to medical treatment for steroidal rosacea-like dermatitis but was bothered by persistent erythema and pigmentation. Although botulinum toxin therapy was performed for aesthetic reasons, it contributed to almost complete resolution of the erythema at two-week follow-up and complete disappearance without recurrence after six months.

For more information about the dermal effects of botulinum toxin therapy, see the *Botulinum Toxin in Cosmetic Dermatology & Skincare Practice* book.

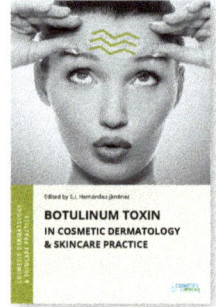

Chapter 9
Diet in rosacea

9.1. Food triggers

The clinical manifestation of rosacea can depend on a variety of external and internal factors, including nutrition (Weiss E., Katta R., 2017). Certain foods are known to cause worsening of the disease, but information offered in publications on this topic is often contradictory.

Alcohol

The most potent triggers for rosacea manifestation and exacerbation are alcoholic beverages, namely wine (red wine has been reported to be a more potent trigger than white wine). As a part of their large-scale study (n = 82,737) Li S. et al. (2017) examined the effect of alcohol consumption on the incidence of rosacea during a 14-year period. The authors noted a significantly higher incidence of rosacea in the group (n = 4945) that reported higher alcohol consumption.

Presumably, the breakdown of acetaldehyde and acetone (metabolites of alcohol) produces histamine, causing dermal vasodilation and facial redness. An additional mechanism of alcohol-induced hyperemia is related to the opiate-like action of enkephalin.

Unfermented tea

According to Wang B. et al. (2021), a higher risk of rosacea is associated with the type of tea (unfermented tea in particular), frequency of daily consumption (≥3 times/day), temperature (60 °C or above), tea strength (>5 g), and total monthly consumption (≥125 g).

Presumably, because of the high concentration of polyphenols (especially catechins) in unfermented tea, the vasodilatory effects may outweigh the anti-inflammatory and antioxidant effects, thereby increasing the risk of rosacea. Based on these results, rosacea patients are advised to consume fermented tea, reduce daily tea intake, and consume the beverage warm rather than hot (Wang B. et al., 2021).

Caffeine

It was previously thought that drinking caffeinated beverages led to the manifestation and aggravation of rosacea symptoms. However, more recent studies have restored the "reputation" of caffeine, as neither water nor coffee was found to cause redness when consumed at temperatures below 22 °C. Erythema occurs after drinking hot beverages (at 60 °C or above). It appears that the high temperature of the beverage, not the type of beverage, is the main trigger. Hot beverages are thought to increase vasodilation and activate the sympathetic nervous system, leading to hyperemia and telangiectasias (Bray E.R. et al., 2020; Searle T. et al., 2021).

In a study conducted by Li S. et al. (2018) involving 4,945 patients, the effect of caffeine consumption on the incidence of rosacea was evaluated. The authors found a clear inverse association between the risk of rosacea and caffeine, with higher caffeine intake associated with a lower incidence of rosacea. Apparently, caffeine has a vasoconstrictive effect, reducing rosacea symptoms.

Niacin-rich food

Niacin (nicotinic acid, vitamin B_3) may be partly responsible for the redness flashes. It is found in salmon, peanuts, tuna, liver, and chicken breasts. Niacin binds to Langerhans cell receptors, releasing prostaglandins around capillaries, leading to erythema, increased skin temperature, itching, and burning (Searle T. et al., 2021).

Spicy food

According to a 400-patient survey conducted by the US National Rosacea Society, after eliminating capsaicin-containing spices, hot sauce, cayenne pepper, and red pepper from the diet, 75% of respondents experienced a reduction in rosacea exacerbations. Regarding the trigger mechanism, vasodilation and redness were attributed to capsaicin activation of TRPV1 receptors by Searle T. et al. (2021).

Cinnamaldehyde

Cinnamaldehyde is found in tomatoes, citrus fruits, and chocolate. According to the research conducted by the US National Rosacea Society, cinnamaldehyde activates the TRPA1 receptors of the sensory nerves of the dermis. As a result, vasodilation, edema, erythema, and telangiectasias develop (Searle T. et al., 2021).

Histamine-rich food

Foods high in histamine (e.g., aged cheese, sauerkraut, wine, and fried meats) can act as triggers for worsening rosacea symptoms. Histamine released by mast cells causes increased vascular permeability, tissue edema, blood flow, and endothelial barrier dysfunction. These effects are particularly pronounced in individuals that have histamine intolerance, which may be caused by an imbalance between the level of absorbed histamine and the ability of the body to break it down (Searle T. et al., 2021).

Fatty food

A diet high in fatty foods (e.g., fatty meats, fried foods, and lard) is associated with a higher risk of rosacea. Fatty foods contribute to chronic inflammation and can also cause an imbalance in the synthesis of ceramides and hyaluronic acid and a relative deficiency of short-chain fatty acids. Consequently, the epidermal barrier is disrupted, and epidermal nerve fibers (C-type) are elongated. This can lead to rosacea symptoms such as pain, burning, and tingling (Searle T. et al., 2021).

Dairy products

Available data on the effect of dairy products on the pathogenesis of rosacea are contradictory. On the one hand, dairy products may have anti-inflammatory properties and contribute to the normalization of the gut microbiome. On the other hand, dairy products cause inflammation and exacerbate the manifestations of acne. Since acne and rosacea have similar pathophysiology, it is unclear how dairy products can have opposite effects on these diseases. Therefore, more in-depth research is needed to reach a definitive conclusion (Searle T. et al., 2021).

9.2. Nutrients indicated for patients with rosacea

Several food substances have been found to have a positive impact on the skin affected by rosacea. The beneficial impact is realized by strengthening the skin barrier and normalizing immunity.

9.2.1. Supporting the skin's defense mechanisms

Omega-3 unsaturated fatty acids

Promising results yielded by several studies suggest the benefits of omega-3 fatty acids for patients affected by rosacea. Omega-3 fatty acids are polyunsaturated fatty acids, which include eicosapentaenoic acid, docosahexaenoic acid, and α-linolenic acid. Because eicosapentaenoic and docosahexaenoic acid are substrates for anti-inflammatory prostaglandins that competitively inhibit inflammatory responses, they have been studied in the context of many diseases (Maroon J.C., Bost J.W., 2006).

For example, Bhargava R. et al. (2013) found statistically significant symptom improvements in patients with dry eye syndrome (dry keratoconjunctivitis), some of whom also suffered from rosacea. The patients took 325 mg of eicosapentaenoic acid and 175 mg of docosahexaenoic acid twice a day for three months.

Zinc

Zinc is involved in cell-mediated innate immunity and has antioxidant and anti-inflammatory properties (Prasad A.S., 2009). However, studies on the effectiveness of zinc preparations in rosacea have produced contradictory results. For example, Sharquie K.E. et al. (2006) noted significant improvements with 100 mg of zinc sulfate administered three times daily. On the other hand, Bamford J.T.M. et al. (2012) reported no benefits of taking 220 mg of zinc sulfate twice a day in alleviating the rosacea patients' symptoms at 90-day follow-up.

9.2.2. Restoring the balance of the intestinal microbiome

The composition of gut bacteria has been postulated to play a role in the pathogenesis of rosacea (Chen Y.J. et al., 2020). Some experts believe that altering the "healthy" composition of the gut microbiome leads to systemic activation of kallikrein–kinin pathways and the development of neurogenic inflammation (Weiss E., Katta R., 2017). In this regard, restoring the balance of the intestinal microbiome is one of the directions of rosacea treatment.

Prebiotics
Basic recommendations for a healthy gut microbiome include eating fiber-rich foods. Ample body of evidence indicates that including a variety of dietary fiber in the daily diet in sufficient quantities promotes the growth of saprophytic ("good") intestinal bacteria (El Kaoutari A. et al., 2013). On the other hand, the absence of dietary fiber is associated with harmful effects on the microflora of the digestive tract and the gastrointestinal tract itself.

In mice fed with food with a low amount of dietary fiber, there was a rapid growth of pathogenic microorganisms, which after some time began to digest the protective mucous layer of the digestive tract. Conversely, a diet rich in dietary fiber supported the growth of beneficial bacteria (Hill C. et al., 2014; Desai M.S. et al., 2016).

Probiotics
The activity of beneficial microorganisms in the digestive tract can be supported by a diet rich in probiotics — fermented foods in which live microbial communities are a leading component (yogurt, kefir, miso, kimchi, and sauerkraut). Several probiotics have been developed and are sold in retail stores in some countries. They can be added to any food to enrich it with beneficial bacteria. However, some researchers believe that such supplements contain low amounts of microorganisms while lacking the diversity of microflora needed for improving the gut microbiome (Scourboutakos M.J. et al., 2017).

Despite positive results of probiotic use in patients affected by inflammatory skin diseases, clinical trials involving rosacea-affected cohorts are lacking. Further studies are thus needed to determine the optimal dosage and selection of specific microbial strains and to ascertain their viability.

Several possible mechanisms underlying the probiotics' potential beneficial effect on rosacea have been suggested (Weiss E., Katta R., 2017).

First, these drugs alter the composition of the gastrointestinal microbiome and help fight pathogenic bacteria. Several studies have demonstrated attenuation of T-cell-mediated skin inflammation in mice after administration of oral probiotics (Hacini-Rachinel F. et al., 2009; Kober M., Bowe W.P., 2015).

Second, *in vitro* incubation of metabolites of a particular bacterial strain has been shown to prevent spontaneous and stress-induced ROS formation (Benson K.F. et al., 2012).

Third, probiotics can positively affect the skin, given that they improved the epidermal barrier function and reduced skin sensitivity in the volunteers that took part in the study conducted by Gueniche A., Benyacoub J., et al. (2010).

While these findings are highly informative, further studies on the clinical use of probiotics in rosacea are required.

9.3. Preventing the cardiovascular disorders

The association between cardiovascular and chronic inflammatory diseases such as rheumatoid arthritis and psoriasis has been described in the literature (Hanna A., Frangogiannis N.G., 2020). Individuals affected by psoriasis are thus advised to make dietary modifications to reduce the risk of comorbidities, which has been established in several studies involving patients with rosacea (Li Y. et al., 2020; Tsai T.Y. et al., 2020; Choi D. et al., 2021).

As previously noted, patients with rosacea have an increased risk of cardiovascular diseases and metabolic disorders. Cathelicidin peptide and serine proteases are thought to act as etiopathogenetic agents in both rosacea and atherosclerosis, but whether these processes can be influenced by diet remains to be determined.

9.4. General recommendations

Based on the available research findings and accumulated clinical evidence, the following general recommendations have been formulated for rosacea patients (Weiss E., Katta R., 2017; rosacea.org):

1. Use with caution or avoid hot drinks, alcohol, foods containing capsaicin (peppers, spices, hot sauces), cinnamaldehyde (cinnamon, chocolate, tomatoes, and citrus fruits), histamine (fermented foods and beverages — wine, beer, vermouth, cider, and vinegar; certain oriental foods; processed beef and pork; and canned fish such as anchovies, tuna, herring, mackerel, and sardines).
2. Add to your daily diet foods with live bacterial cultures (yogurt, kefir, sauerkraut), and prebiotics (inulin, dietary fiber).
3. Consume foods rich in omega-3 fatty acids:
   - Vegetable oils: flaxseed oil, rapeseed oil, soybean oil, corn oil, olive oil, sesame oil, wheat germ oil
   - Fish: mackerel, sardines, herring, salmon, tuna, trout, catfish, etc.
   - Seafood: mussels, squid, shrimp, crab, scallops, cod liver, pollock roe, black caviar, wakame seaweed, oysters
   - Nuts: walnuts, pine nuts, almonds, pistachios, pecans, cashews
   - Butternut pumpkin, pumpkin seeds
   - Soybeans, soy milk
   - Eggs, camembert cheese, tofu
   - Avocado, spinach, broccoli, cauliflower, Brussels sprouts, greens (dill, parsley, portulaca, cilantro)
4. Consume foods rich in zinc (despite some conflicting research results, they at least do not worsen the rosacea manifestation): oysters, wheat bran, fried veal liver, cooked eels, beef stew, sesame seeds, pumpkin seeds, cooked chicken hearts, pine nuts.

Part II

Couperosis

Chapter 1
Etiology

Couperosis is a non-inflammatory skin pathology characterized by persistent dilation of small skin vessels and multiple telangiectasias (**Fig. II-1-1**).

It is difficult to identify the exact causes of couperosis, but several factors are known to provoke its development, as outlined below.

1. Genetic predisposition: telangiectasias are more likely to occur in people with fair skin.
2. Sun exposure: UV damage to the skin is one of the leading causes of facial telangiectasias. UVA radiation, which can reach the dermis blood vessels, mediates direct and indirect damage to cells and dermal structures, triggering oxidative stress, activation of MMP synthesis, and destruction of connective tissue (including vessel walls). In addition, UV action

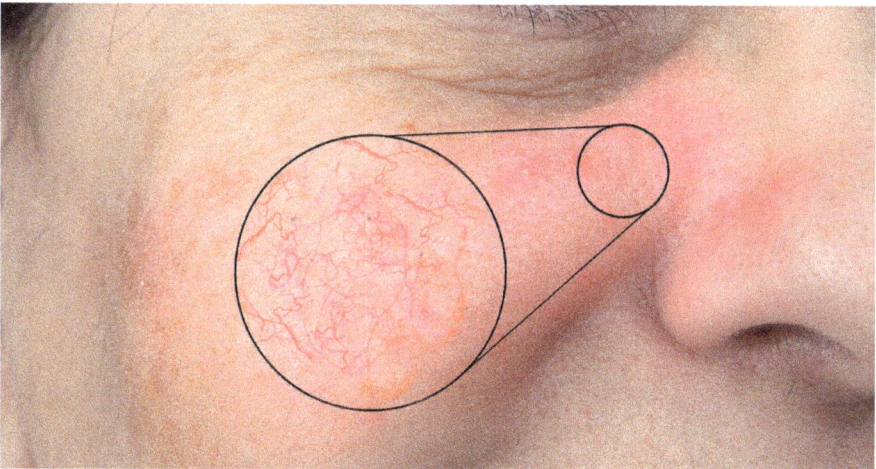

Figure II-1-1. Couperose on the nose and cheek
(Image by Alessandro Grandini, Freepik.com)

leads to vascular dilation, which, along with structural changes, gradually becomes persistent.

3. Exposure to wind and temperature variations
4. Use of some medications:
   - Vasodilators, especially calcium channel blockers (sun-exposed areas are mainly affected)
   - Long-acting systemic corticosteroids
   - Long-acting topical corticosteroids (including the development of the steroidal rosacea)
   - Intralesional injections of triamcinolone
5. Pregnancy
6. Hypertension
7. Acne
8. Weight gain
9. Drinking too much alcohol
10. Smoking
11. Skin damage, including surgical trauma
12. Aggressive aesthetic treatments

Hormone therapy and hormonal changes due to menopause or taking birth-control pills can also lead to the formation of facial telangiectasias. Older people are also more likely to develop telangiectasia, as blood vessels weaken with age.

Chapter 2
Clinical manifestation

Telangiectasias are permanently dilated small skin vessels (capillaries, venules, arterioles) 0.1–1 mm in diameter, making them visible to the naked eye. Capillary telangiectasias are pink-red, arteriolar are intensely red, while venular are blue-violet in color. Unlike capillary and arteriolar, venular telangiectasias are usually elevated above the skin surface.

Dilated vessels can be located at the subepidermal level (superficial telangiectasias in photoaging) as well as at the dermal level (deep secondary telangiectasias in severe photoaging, age-related telangiectasias, telangiectasias in rosacea, collagenosis). The diameter of superficial vessels is smaller than that of deep ones.

Externally, telangiectasias may look like vascular asterisks (many vascular branches diverge from the central part raised above the skin) or meshes (scattered vessels), as shown in **Fig. II-2-1**. They become pale when pressure is applied. In couperosis, the most typical localization of telangiectasias is on the wings of the nose, cheeks, and chin. In most cases, telangiectasias do not cause any unpleasant sensations. However, sometimes they may bleed.

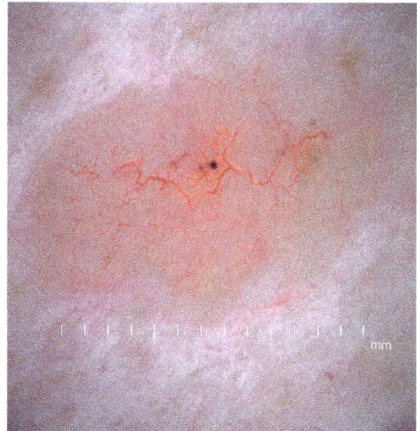

Figure II-2-1. Telangiectasia (Image by David.moreno72, Wikipedia)

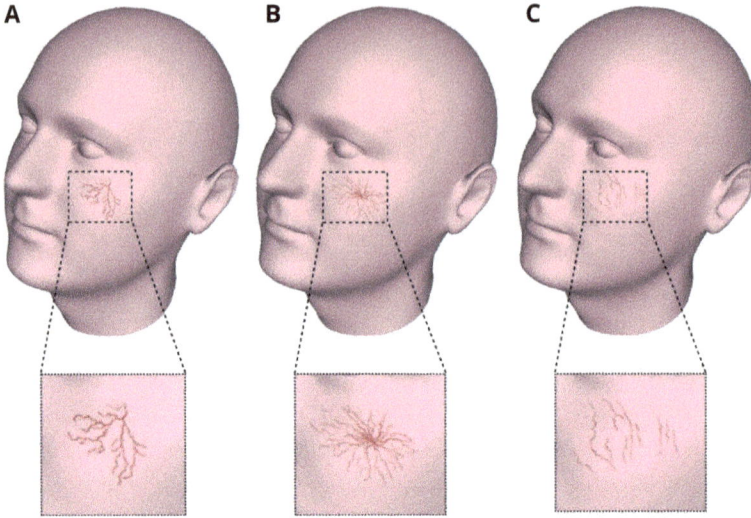

Figure II-2-2. Types of telangiectasias: (A) arborizing, (B) spider, and (C) linear (adapted from Liapakis E.L. et al., 2015)

There are three types of telangiectasias (**Fig. II-2-2**) (Liapakis E.L. et al., 2015):
1. Simple, linear
2. Arborizing (branch-like)
3. Spider (cartwheel shaped with a central point)

Some experts also recognize a 4th type: spotted telangiectasias — a cluster of many tiny dots on the skin that are more often a symptom of other diseases.

In the formation of couperosis, four stages are described:
- Stage 1: the appearance of barely visible dilated capillaries on the background of temporary redness (with high temperature, excitement) or irritation of the skin of the face.
- Stage 2: dilated capillaries gradually merge into a mesh, the vessels' color becomes more visible to the naked eye.
- Stage 3: the appearance of persistent telangiectasias, mainly in the central third of the face.
- Stage 4: visible vascular stars and mesh, widespread throughout the face. Areas of local pallor may be formed due to microcirculation disorders and capillary spasms.

Chapter 3
Diagnostics

The diagnosis of facial couperosis is simple, as the presence of telangiectasias on the face is the sole criterion. While these manifestations are usually accompanied by no other symptoms, people with couperosis sometimes experience skin hypersensitivity. Still, this is more of a parallel process than a consequence of vascular disorders.

Although there are many diseases in which telangiectasias are observed, the differential diagnosis of couperosis is usually made with **erythematotelangiectatic rosacea**. These conditions are often confused because telangiectasias are a symptom of rosacea, but can be associated with other conditions with distinct symptomology (**Table II-3-1**).

Table II-3-1. Couperosis *vs*. erythematotelangiectatic rosacea

FACIAL COUPEROSIS	ERYTHEMATOTELANGIECTATIC RO-SACEA
Telangiectasias are more often localized on the wings of the nose, cheeks, and chin	Telangiectasias can be located anywhere
No gender segregation	More frequently seen in women
No symptoms of inflammation	There are symptoms of inflammation
No or minimal erythema flare-ups, lasting less than 10 minutes	Erythema flare-ups are present, lasting more than 10 minutes
The skin is more likely to be calm	Sensitive skin

Telangiectasias may also be observed in individuals affected by connective tissue diseases such as localized scleroderma (telangiectasias against the background of atrophic processes in the skin) and dermatomyositis (as a part of the musculoskeletal system disorder). Both diseases are characterized by telangiectasias not only on the face but also on other parts of the body, especially near nail phalanges. Another cause may be **liver pathology**.

Chapter 4
Treating couperosis

Since couperosis is accompanied by structural changes in the blood vessel walls, topical therapeutic and cosmetic agents are ineffective in its treatment. The main treatment options are related to the destruction of vessels by energy-based devices. However, several preventive and therapeutic measures may help slow the disease progression.

4.1. Lifestyle

Lifestyle recommendations for patients with couperosis are similar to those for individuals affected by rosacea but are less strict. Nonetheless, the following recommendations should be followed:

- Protecting your skin from the sun with sunscreen, clothing, hat, and shade
- Minimizing exposure to excessively high or low temperatures and other triggers of vascular dilation (spicy and hot food, physical activity, etc.), rough mechanical impact, and skin damage from aggressive cosmetic procedures
- Limiting the use of topical steroids

To date, no recommended topical remedies, either pharmacological or cosmetic, have proven effective in eliminating couperosis. However, taking care of the skin with couperosis is essential both to strengthen it and to slow down the development of the disease.

4.2. Cosmetic care for couperosis

4.2.1 Skin cleansing

Recommendations for cleansing the skin with couperosis are also similar to those for rosacea:
- Use mild products free from alcohol, detergents, abrasives
- Wash out with room temperature water. "Training vessels" with hot and cold water and wiping with ice can aggravate couperosis
- No intensive mechanical impact (no abrasion or stretching)
- Acid peels and (micro)dermabrasion are not recommended. Enzymatic peels are allowed

4.2.2. Home care

The main purpose of home care should be moisturizing and protection. Care products should not contain aggressive components. Hot masks and intensive facial massage are not recommended. Light lymphatic drainage massage is possible as a congestion prevention.

4.2.3. Cosmetic ingredients with vasoconstrictive properties

Some cosmetic ingredients can slow down (but not block!) the couperosis progression:
- Vitamins K, PP, E, C
- Rutin
- Arnica extract
- Horse chestnut extract
- Nettle extract
- Ivy extract
- Centella extract
- Green tea extract
- Ginkgo biloba extract
- Bilberry extract

4.2.4. Cosmetic camouflage

A flesh-colored foundation can conceal mild telangiectasia. a foundation or moisturizer with a greenish tint is preferable for more prominent telangiectasias and facial redness. Such a product is usually marketed as "concealer," "redness remover," or "anti-redness."

Chapter 5
Injection treatment

Unlike rosacea, couperosis can be treated with injectables. Some experts recommend mesotherapy to inject the same vasodilating substances as those mentioned earlier. However, microneedling can provoke the formation of telangiectasias.

Another injectable method is micro-sclerotherapy which involves the injection of drugs that "glue" the vessels together (ethoxysclerol, sodium tetradecyl sulfate, etc.), usually to remove telangiectasias on the legs. This procedure is challenging in facial capillary telangiectasias because the vessels are tiny, making it difficult to insert the needle into them. However, it can be used for large "blue" telangiectasias resulting from venules. The best results are achieved with vessels exceeding 0.4 mm in diameter. It is also important to note that, in the case of sclerotherapy of capillary and arteriolar telangiectasias with a diameter below 0.2 mm, a complication in the form of necrosis of the overlying skin is possible (Goldman M.P., Bergan J.J., 2001). For facial telangiectasias, use of glycerin as a sclerosant is advised (McGregor S. et al., 2019).

Like in sclerotherapy of vessels on the legs, some experts suggest using silicone patches to increase the effectiveness of sclerotherapy on the face (Misirlioglu A. et al., 2004).

In general, sclerotherapy on the face is undesirable because of the likelihood of the subsequent formation of uneven skin texture at the sclerosing site.

Chapter 6
Energy-based therapy

6.1. Electrical methods

6.1.1. Microcurrent therapy

Microcurrent therapy relies on the application of modulated pulsed direct currents of very low intensity (in the microampere range, 1 μA = 1/1,000,000 A) with different frequency characteristics for medical and aesthetic purposes. Microcurrents influence the arterioles' smooth muscle cells, changing the vascular wall's tone. Thus, microcurrent stimulation improves skin microcirculation. This method can be used for couperosis prevention by improving the tone of blood vessels, but not as therapy because microcurrents cannot eliminate the existing telangiectasia.

6.1.2. Electrocoagulation and RF microneedling

Electrocoagulation involves application of a high-frequency alternating electric current for local tissue heating with the aim of their thermal destruction (cauterization).

For coagulation of vessels in couperosis or telangiectasia, a hair electrode conducting a low current (1–2 A) is used. Cauterizations are made at 2–3 mm distance from each other. It is essential to remove the supplying vessel, which automatically eliminates the vascular defect. However, this is not always possible, because the vascular network in couperosis is most often branched, without clear boundaries and a single source of supply. Sometimes, several sessions may be required (Goldman M.P., 2004). After electrocoagulation, the formation of pigmented defects and scarring is possible.

Another option for eliminating telangiectasias is RF microneedling, as its mechanism of action for couperosis will be similar (see Part I, section 7.2).

6.2. Light therapy

The mechanism of action of light radiation in couperosis elimination is based on the selective photothermolysis effect, as described in detail in the part devoted to light therapy for rosacea (see Part I, section 7.1).

Telangiectasias are a very convenient target for laser and IPL devices because dilated vessels contain a small but increased number of red blood cells carrying hemoglobin, a primary target for light. Therefore, hemoglobin simply transfers the energy that will lead to thermolysis of the vascular wall (coagulation or rupture, depending on the pulse duration).

Superficial telangiectasias are faster and easier to treat with IPL, KTR, and PDL devices emitting pulses of short duration. Deep telangiectasias have a larger caliber, which requires an extended pulse mode, high energy density, large spots, and longer wavelengths.

Table II-6-1 summarizes the main types of devices currently used to treat various telangiectasias (Sheptii O.V., 2018).

Surface cooling during the session reduces the risk of thermal damage and discomfort. Cooling is particularly important when using shorter-wavelength lasers (KTP, PDL).

Light therapy administered through 1–3 sessions is effective in 60–90% of cases (Sheptii O.V., 2018). It is the most effective method for fighting couperosis although, in many cases, pathologically altered vessels tend to reoccur.

6.3. Cryodestruction

Cryodestruction is a method of bloodless destruction of pathological tissue by short-term freezing by exposing it to ultra-low temperatures with subsequent tissue elimination. Freezing is accompanied by a hemostatic effect due to the disruption of microcirculation in capillaries.

Table II-6-1. Devices for treating different types of telangiectasias (Sheptii O.V., 2018)

DEVICE	TARGET / DEPTH	DISADVANTAGES
KTR laser, λ = 532 nm (green)	Oxyhemoglobin > melanin; 1 mm	Usually used for more superficial vessels Marked epidermal damage in dark-skinned people (dyschromia and textural changes, sometimes scarring)
PDL laser, λ = 585–595 nm (yellow)	Oxyhemoglobin > melanin; 1–1.5 mm	Pain, purpura (especially with short pulse and high energy density) Like the KTP laser, it is mainly used for more superficial vessels
IPL, λ = 500–1200 nm	Filters for vascular lesions at λ = 550 and 570 nm (yellow and green light)	Pain, heat burns, dyschromia It is difficult to establish reliable treatment parameters due to the many differences in devices

During cryoexposure, pathological tissue is not removed, but gradually necrotized, and the upper necrotized layer acts as an antiseptic dressing, providing complete organotypic healing without forming keloid scars and undesirable aesthetic defects. Cryodestruction is indicated in tuberous, cavernous, and stellate hemangiomas.

The frozen tissue becomes white, cold, dense, and insensitive, with sensations of slight burning, tingling, and slight pain. Within the first three hours, hyperemia and collateral edema develop, and after 6–24 hours, epidermal blisters (with serous or hemorrhagic contents) appear. As a rule, the blister is not opened, but if it is painful and large, it should be opened and treated with Brilliant green or Castellani paint. After 2–6 weeks, the necrosis zone is wholly rejected, leaving barely noticeable pink spot as a result of the epithelization of the defect and the surrounding tissue. All elements and structures of the dermis are restored within 3–6 months.

Afterwords

Rosacea and couperosis seem to have similar pathologies, even though their causes are different. Both conditions involve blood vessels, but couperosis is linked to structural changes, whereas rosacea is primarily a functional disorder caused by a vast number of pathogenetic factors, although telangiectasias are also present.

Another common feature is progression, as both processes usually worsen over time. Still, if couperosis can be regarded as an aesthetic defect, rosacea is a disease that significantly influences the quality of life. Many triggers can provoke rosacea progression, which leads to manifestations that are increasingly disfiguring.

The good news is that aesthetic medicine offers solutions that, while not leading to a permanent cure, can significantly slow the disease progression and help patients achieve remission. That means not just looking better but living better.

We hope that the information we have presented in this book will help you build an optimal therapeutic course for rosacea and couperosis, and significantly facilitate the life of your clients with these pathologies.

References

Ahn C.S., Huang W.W. Rosacea pathogenesis. Dermatol Clin 2018; 36(2): 81–86.

Ahn T.H., Cho S.B. Invasive pulsed-type, bipolar, alternating current radiofrequency treatment using microneedle electrodes for nasal rosacea. Med Lasers 2017; 6(1): 32–36.

Anderson R.R., Parrish J.A. Selective photothermolysis: precise micro-surgery by selective absorption of pulsed radiation. Science 1983; 220(4596): 524–527.

Aşiran Serdar Z., Aktaş Karabay E. a case of fractional microneedling radiofrequency induced rosacea. J Cosmet Laser Ther 2019; 21(6): 349–351.

Atiakshin D., Buchwalow I., Tiemann M. Mast cells and collagen fibrillogenesis. Histochem Cell Biol 2020; 154(1): 21–40.

Aubdool A.A., Brain S.D. Neurovascular aspects of skin neurogenic inflammation. J Invest Dermatol Symp Proc 2011; 15(1): 33–39.

Bamford J.T.M., Gessert C.E., Haller I.V., et al. Randomized, double-blind trial of 220 mg zinc sulfate twice daily in rosacea treatment. Int J Dermatol 2012; 51(4): 459–462.

Bansal C., Omlin K.J., Hayes C.M., Rohrer T.E. Novel cutaneous uses for botulinum toxin type A. J Cosmet Dermatol 2006; 5 (3): 268–272.

Baylie R.L., Brayden J.E. TRPV channels and vascular function. Acta Physiol (Oxf) 2011; 203(1): 99–116.

Beck-Speier I., Oswald B., Maier K.L. et al. Oxymetazoline inhibits and resolves inflammatory reactions in human neutrophils. J Pharmacol Sci 2009; 110(3): 276–284.

Benson K.F., Redman K.A., Carter S.G. et al. Probiotic metabolites from Bacillus coagulans GanedenBC30TM support maturation of antigen-presenting cells in vitro. World J Gastroenterol 2012; 18(16): 1875–1883.

Bhargava R., Kumar P., Kumar M. et al. a randomized controlled trial of omega-3 fatty acids in dry eye syndrome. Int J Ophthalmol 2013; 6(6): 811–816.

Bharti J., Sonthalia S., Jakhar D. Mesotherapy with Botulinum toxin for the treatment of refractory vascular and papulopustular rosacea 2023; 88(6): e295–e296.

Bielenberg D.R., Bucana C.D., Sanchez R. et al. Molecular regulation of UVB-induced cutaneous angiogenesis. J Invest Dermatol 1998; 111(5): 864–872.

Blanchet-Réthoré S., Bourdès V., Mercenier A. et al. Effect of a lotion containing the heat-treated probiotic strain Lactobacillus johnsonii NCC 533 on Staphylococcus aureus colonization in atopic dermatitis. Clin Cosmet Invest Dermatol 2017; 10: 249–257.

Bloom B.S., Payongayong L., Mourin A., Goldberg D.J. Impact of intradermal abobotulinumtoxinA on facial erythema of rosacea. Dermatol Surg 2015; 41(1): 9–16.

Bray E.R., Kirsner R.S., Issa N.T. Coffee and skin — Considerations beyond the caffeine perspective. J Am Acad Dermatol 2020; 82(2): e63.

Brown M., O'Reilly S. The immunopathogenesis of fibrosis in systemic sclerosis. Clin Exp Immunol 2019; 195(3): 310–321.

Buddenkotte J., Steinhoff M. Recent advances in understanding and managing rosacea. F1000Res 2018; 7: F1000 Faculty Rev-1885.

Buhl T., Sulk M., Nowak P. et al. Molecular and morphological characterization of inflammatory infiltrate in rosacea reveals activation of Th1/Th17 pathways. J Invest Dermatol 2015; 135(9): 2198–2208.

Campolmi P., Bonan P., Cannarozzo C. et al. Highlights of thirty-year experience of CO_2 laser use at the Florence (Italy) Department of Dermatology. Sci World J 2012; 2012: 546528.

Carmichael N.M., Dostrovsky J.O., Charlton M.P. Peptide-mediated transdermal delivery of botulinum neurotoxin type a reduces neurogenic inflammation in the skin. Pain 2010; 149(2): 316–324.

Casas M.N., Monaco M., Magliano J., Bazzano C. Hard-to-diagnose unilateral facial dermatosis. Clin Case Rep J 2020; 1(5): 1–3.

Celiker H., Toker E., Ergun T., Cinel L. An unusual presentation of ocular rosacea. Arquivos Brasileiros de Oftalmologia 2017; 80(6): 396–398.

Chang A.L.S., Raber I., Xu J. et al. Assessment of the genetic basis of rosacea by genome-wide association study. Invest Dermatol 2015; 135(6): 1548–1555.

Chen Y.J., Lee W.H., Ho H.J. et al. An altered fecal microbial profiling in rosacea patients compared to matched controls. J Formos Med Assoc 2020; 120(1 Pt 1): 256–264.

Chhabra G., Garvey D.R., Singh C.K. et al. Effects and mechanism of nicotinamide against UVA-and/or UVB-mediated DNA damages in normal melanocytes. Photochem Photobiol 2019; 95(1): 331–337.

Choi D., Choi S., Choi S. et al. Association of rosacea with cardiovascular disease: a retrospective cohort study. J Am Heart Assoc 2021; 10(19): e020671.

Choi J.E., Werbel T., Wang Z. et al. Botulinum toxin blocks mast cells and prevents rosacea like inflammation. J Dermatol Sci 2019; 93(1): 58–64.

Chosidow O., Cribier B. Epidemiology of rosacea: updated data. Ann Dermatol Venereol 2011; 138(Suppl 3): 179–83.

Dai Y., Wang S., Tominaga M. et al. Sensitization of TRPA1 by PAR2 contributes to the sensation of inflammatory pain. J Clin Invest 2007; 117(7): 1979–1987.

Dayan S.H., Ashourian N., Cho K. a pilot, double-blind, placebo-controlled study to assess the efficacy and safety of incobotulinumtoxinA injections in the treatment of rosacea. J Drugs Dermatol 2017; 16(6): 549–554.

Delinasios G.J., Karbaschi M., Cooke M.S. Young A.R. Vitamin E inhibits the UVAI induction of "light" and "dark" cyclobutane pyrimidine dimers, and oxidatively generated DNA damage, in keratinocytes. Sci Rep. 2018; 8(1): 423.

Del Rosso J.Q. Advances in understanding and managing rosacea: part 1: connecting the dots between pathophysiological mechanisms and common clinical features of rosacea with emphasis on vascular changes and facial erythema. J Clin Aesthet Dermatol 2012; 5(3): 16–25.

Del Rosso J.Q., Thiboutot D., Gallo R. et al. American Acne & Rosacea Society. Consensus recommendations from the American Acne & amp; Rosacea Society on the management of rosacea, part 5: a guide on the management of rosacea. Cutis 2014; 93(3): 134–138.

Deng Z., Chen M., Zhao Z. et al. Whole genome sequencing identifies genetic variants associated with neurogenic inflammation in rosacea. Nat Commun 2023; 14(1): 3958.

Desai M.S., Seekatz A.M., Koropatkin N.M. et al. a dietary fiber-deprived gut microbiota degrades the colonic mucus barrier and enhances pathogen susceptibility. Cell 2016; 167(5): 1339–1353.

Diaz C., O'Callaghan C.J., Khan A., Ilchyshyn A. Rosacea: a cutaneous marker of Helicobacter pylori infection? Results of a pilot study. Acta Derm Venereol 2003; 83(4): 282–286.

Diffey B. Sunscreen claims, risk management and consumer confidence. Int J Cosmet Sci 2020; 42(1): 1–4.

Draelos Z.D., Ertel K., Berge C. Niacinamide-containing facial moisturizer improves skin barrier and benefits subjects with rosacea. Cutis 2005; 76 (2): 135–141.

Drago F., De Col E., Agnoletti A.F. et al. The role of small intestinal bacterial overgrowth in rosacea: a 3-year follow-up. J Am Acad Dermatol 2016; 75(3): 113–115.

Egeberg A., Weinstock L.B., Thyssen E.P. et al. Rosacea and gastrointestinal disorders: a population-based cohort study. Br J Dermatol 2017; 176(1): 100–106.

El Kaoutari A., Armougom F., Gordon J.I. et al. The abundance and variety of carbohydrate-active enzymes in the human gut microbiota. Nat Rev Microbiol 2013; 11(7): 497–504.

Ferrer L., Ravera I., Silbermayr K. Immunology and pathogenesis of canine demodicosis. Vet Dermatol 2014; 25(5): 427–465.

Forbat E., Al-Niaimi F., Ali F.R. The emerging importance of tranexamic acid in dermatology. Clin Exp Dermatol 2020; 45(4): 445–449.

Friedman O., Koren A., Niv R. et al. The toxic edge-A novel treatment for refractory erythema and flushing of rosacea. Lasers Surg Med 2019; 51(4): 325–331.

Gallo R.L, Granstein R.D., Kang S. et al. Standard classification and pathophysiology of rosacea: The 2017 update by the National Rosacea Society Expert Committee. J Am Acad Dermatol 2018; 78(1): 148–155.

Gammoh N.Z., Rink L. Zinc in infection and inflammation. Nutrients 2017; 9(6): 624.

Gether L., Overgaard L.K., Egeberg A., Thyssen J.P. Incidence and prevalence of rosacea: a systematic review and meta-analysis. Br J Dermatol 2018; 179(2): 282–289.

Giacalone S., Minuti A., Spigariolo C.B. et al. Facial dermatoses in the general population due to wearing of personal protective masks during the COVID-19 pandemic: first observations after lockdown. Clin Exp Dermatol 2021; 46(2): 368–369.

Goldberg D. (ed.). Lasers and Lights. Sounders/Elsevier, 2007.

Goldman M.P. Optimal management of facial telangiectasia. Am J Clin Dermatol 2004; 5(6): 423–434.

Goldman M.P., Bergan J.J. Sclerotherapy treatment of varicose and telangiectatic leg veins. 3rd ed. St Louis (MO): Harcourt Health Sciences, 2001.

Graepel R., Fernandes E.S., Aubdool A.A. et al. 4-oxo-2-nonenal (4-ONE): evidence of transient receptor potential ankyrin 1-dependent and -independent nociceptive and vasoactive responses in vivo. J Pharmacol Exp Ther 2011; 337(1): 117–124.

Gravina A., Federico A., Ruocco E. et al. Helicobacter pylori infection but not small intestinal bacterial overgrowth may play a pathogenic role in rosacea. Un Eur Gastroenterol J 2015; 3(1): 17–24.

Guéniche A., Bastien P., Ovigne J.M. et al. Bifidobacterium longum lysate, a new ingredient for reactive skin. Exp Dermatol 2010; 19(8): 1–8.

Guéniche A., Benyacoub J., Philippe D. et al. Lactobacillus paracasei CNCM I-2116 (ST11) inhibits substance P-induced skin inflammation and accelerates skin barrier function recovery in vitro. Eur J Dermatol 2010; 20(6): 731–737.

Gupta V.K., Paul S., Dutta C. Geography, ethnicity or subsistence-specific variations in human microbiome composition and diversity. Front Microbiol 2017; 23(8): 162.

Guzman-Sanchez D.A., Ishiuji Y., Patel T. et al. Enhanced skin blood flow and sensitivity to noxious heat stimuli in papulopustular rosacea. J Am Acad Dermatol 2007; 57(5): 800–805.

Haber R., El Gemayel M. Comorbidities in rosacea: a systematic review and update. J Am Acad Dermatol 2018; 78(4): 786–792. e8.

Hacini-Rachinel F., Gheit H., Le Luduec J.B. et al. Oral probiotic control skin inflammation by acting on both effector and regulatory T cells. PLoS One 2009; 4(3): 4903.

Hanna A., Frangogiannis N.G. Inflammatory cytokines and chemokines as therapeutic targets in heart failure. Cardiovasc Drugs Ther. 2020; 34(6): 849–863.

Harper J. Hot sauce, wine, and tomatoes cause flare-ups, survey finds. In: Rosacea Review by the US National Rosacea Society, 2005. https://shorturl.at/arDV1.

Heisig M., Reich A. Psychosocial aspects of rosacea with a focus on anxiety and depression. Clin Cosmet Invest Dermatol 2018; 11: 103–107.

Hill C., Guarner F., Reid G. et al. Expert consensus document: The International Scientific Association for Probiotics and Prebiotics consensus statement on the scope and appropriate use of the term probiotic. Nat Rev Gastroenterol Hepatol 2014; 11(8): 506–514.

Jackson J.M., Knuckles M., Minni J.P. et al. The role of brimonidine tartrate gel in the treatment of rosacea. Clin Cosmet Invest Dermatol 2015; 8: 529–538.

Kalashnikova N.G. Combined laser correction of keloid scars. Apparatnaya Kosmetologiya & Physiotherapia 2014; 3: 82–86.

Kalashnikova N.G. Practical aspects of scar laser treatment. Cosmetics & Medicine 2016; 3: 64–71.

Kassir R., Gilbreath J., Sajjadian A. Combination surgical excision and fractional carbon dioxide laser for treatment of rhinophyma. World J Plast Surg 2012; 1(1): 36–40.

Katoch S., Barua T.N., Barua K.N. Role of botulinum toxin in the management of topical corticosteroid induced rosacea like dermatitis: a case report. Indian Dermatol Online J 2022; 13(3): 395–397.

Kim J., Chung B., Lee S. et al. Implications of metabolic status on the incidence of rosacea: a Korean nationwide population-based cohort study. 49th Annual ESDR Meeting, Sep 18–21, 2019.

Kim J.Y., Kim Y.J., Lim B.J. et al. Increased expression of cathelicidin by direct activation of protease-activated receptor 2: possible implications on the pathogenesis of rosacea. Yonsei Med J 2014; 55(6): 1648–1655.

Kim M., Kim J., Jeong S.W. et al. Inhibition of mast cell infiltration in an LL-37-induced rosacea mouse model using topical brimonidine tartrate 0.33% gel. Exp Dermatol 2017; 26(11): 1143–1145.

Kiousi D.E., Karapetsas A., Karolidou K. et al. Probiotics in extraintestinal diseases: current trends and new directions. Nutrients 2019; 11(4): 788.

Kligman A.M. a personal critique on the state of knowledge of rosacea. Dermatology 2004; 208(3): 191–197.

Kober M., Bowe W.P. The effect of probiotics on immune regulation, acne, and photoaging. Int J Womens Dermatol 2015; 1(2): 85–89.

Koijak M., Yagli S., Vahapog lu G., Eksioglu M. Permethrin 5% cream versus metronidazole 0.75% gel for the treatment of papulopustular rosacea: a randomized double-blind placebo-controlled study. Dermatology 2002; 205(2–3): 265–270.

Kucher A.N. Neurogenic inflammation: biochemical markers, genetic control, and disease. Bulletin of Siberian Medicine 2020; 19(2): 171–181.

Lasigliè D., Traggiai E., Federici S. et al. Role of IL-1 beta in the development of human T(H)17 cells: lesson from NLPR3 mutated patients. PLoS One 2011; 6(5): 20014.

Li S., Chen M.L., Drucker A.M. et al. Association of caffeine intake and caffeinated coffee consumption with risk of incident rosacea in women. JAMA Dermatol 2018; 154(12): 1394–1400.

Li S., Cho E., Drucker A.M. et al. Alcohol intake and risk of rosacea in US women. J Am Acad Dermatol 2017; 76(6): 1061–1067.

Li W.Q., Cho E., Khalili H. et al. Rosacea, use of tetracycline, and risk of incident inflammatory bowel disease in women. Clin Gastroenterol Hepatol 2016; 14(2): 220–225.

Li Y., Guo L., Hao D., Li X. et al. Association between rosacea and cardiovascular diseases and related risk Ffactors: a systematic review and meta-analysis. Biomed Res Int 2020; 2020: 7015249.

Liapakis E.L., Englander M., Sinani R. et al. Management of facial telangiectasias with hand cautery. World J Plastic Surg 2015; 4(2): 127–133.

Logger J.G.M., Olydam J.I., Driessen R.J.B. Use of beta-blockers for rosacea-associated facial erythema and flushing: a systematic review and update on proposed mode of action. J Am Acad Dermatol 2020; 83(4):1088–1097.

Marek-Jozefowicz L., Nedoszytko B., Grochocka M. et al. Molecular mechanisms of neurogenic inflammation of the skin. Int J Mol Sci 2023; 24(5): 5001.

Maroon J.C., Bost J.W. Omega-3 fatty acids (fish oil) as an anti-inflammatory: an alternative to nonsteroidal anti-inflammatory drugs for discogenic pain. Surg Neurol 2006; 65(4): 326–331.

Marson J.W., Mouser P., Berto S., Baldwin H.E. Cutaneous and enteral dysbiosis: a rosacea pilot study from the Twin's Day Festival. E-poster presented at AAD VMX Virtual Meeting Experience 2020 July 12–14.

Mastrofrancesco A., Ottaviani M., Aspite N., et al. Azelaic acid modulates the inflammatory response in normal human keratinocytes through PPARgamma activation. Exp Dermatol. 2010; 19(9): 813–820.

Maywald M., Wessels I., Rink L. Zinc signals and immunity. Int J Mol Sci 2017; 18(10): 2222.

McGregor S., Miceli A., Krishnamurthy K. Treatment of facial telangiectases with glycerin sclerotherapy. Dermatol Surg 2019; 45(7): 950–953.

Misirlioglu A., Gideroglu K., Akan M., Akoz T. Using silicone gel sheet for the treatment of facial telangiectasias with sclerotherapy. Dermatol Surg 2004; 30(3): 373–377.

Mottin V.H.M., Suyenaga E.S. An approach on the potential use of probiotics in the treatment of skin conditions: acne and atopic dermatitis. Int J Dermatol 2018; 57(12): 1425–1432.

Muizzuddin N., Maher W., Sullivan M. et al. Physiological effect of a probiotic on skin. J Cosmet Sci 2012; 63(6): 385–395.

Muto Y., Wang Z., Vanderberghe M. et al. Mast cells are key mediators of cathelicidin-initiated skin inflammation in rosacea. J Inves Dermatol 2014; 134(11): 2728–2736.

Ní Raghallaigh S., Bender K., Lacey N. et al. The fatty acid profile of the skin surface lipid layer in papulopustular rosacea. Br J Dermatol 2012; 166(2): 279–287.

Ní Raghallaigh S., Powell F.C. Epidermal hydration levels in patients with rosacea improve after minocycline therapy. Br J Dermatol 2014; 171(2): 259–266.

Odo M.E., Odo L.M., Farias R.V. et al. Botulinum toxin for the treatment of menopausal hot flushes: a pilot study. Dermatol Surg 2011; 37(11): 1579–1583.

Okwundu N., Cline A., Feldman S.R. Difference in vasoconstrictors: oxymetazoline vs. brimonidine. J Dermatolog Treat 2019; 32(2): 1–7.

O'Reilly N., Menezes N., Kavanagh K. Positive correlation between serum immunoreactivity to Demodex-associated Bacillus proteins and erythematotelangiectatic rosacea. Br J Dermatol 2012; 167(5): 1032–1036.

Park S.Y., Kwon H.H., Yoon J.Y. et al. Clinical and histologic effects of fractional microneedling radiofrequency treatment on rosacea. Dermatologic Surg 2016; 42(12): 1362–1369.

Plewig G., Kligman A.M. Acne and Rosacea. Springer, 2019.

Pozsgai G., Bodkin J.V., Graepel R. et al. Evidence for the pathophysiological relevance of TRPA1 receptors in the cardiovascular system in vivo. Cardiovasc Res 2010; 87(4): 760–768.

Prasad A.S. Zinc: role in immunity, oxidative stress and chronic inflammation. Curr Opin Clin Nutr Metab Care 2009; 12(6): 646–652.

Rainer B.M., Kang S., Chien A.L. Rosacea: epidemiology, pathogenesis, and treatment. Dermatoendocrinol 2017; 9(1): e1361574.

Rakhanskaya E.M. Pigment disorders: a review of the possibilities of hardware cosmetology. Apparatnaya Kosmetologiya 2016; 3: 6–19.

Rosa A.C., Fantozzi R. The role of histamine in neurogenic inflammation. Br J Pharmacol 2013; 170(1): 38–45.

Say E.M., Gokhan O., Gökdemir G. Treatment outcomes of long-pulsed Nd:YAG laser for two different subtypes of rosacea. Clin Aesthet Dermatol 2015; 8(9): 16–20.

Scala J., Vojvodic A., Vojvodic P. et al. Botulin toxin use in rosacea and facial flushing treatment. Open Access Maced J Med Sci 2019; 7(18): 2985–2987.

Schaller M., Almeida L.M.C., Bewley A. et al. Recommendations for rosacea diagnosis, classification and management: update from the global ROSacea COnsensus 2019 panel. Br J Dermatol 2020; 182(5): 1269–1276.

Scheenstra M.R., van Harten R.M., Veldhuizen E.J.A. et al. Cathelicidins modulate TLR-activation and inflammation. Front Immunol 2020; 11: 1137.

Scheman A., Rakowski E.M., Chou V. et al. Balsam of Peru: past and future. Dermatitis. 2013; 24(4): 153–160.

Scourboutakos M.J., Franco-Arellano B., Murphy S.A. et al. Mismatch between probiotic benefits in trials vs food products. Nutrients 2017; 9(4): 400.

Searle T., Ali F.R., Carolides S., Al-Niaimi F. Rosacea and diet: what is new in 2021? J Clin Aesthet Dermatol 2021; 14(12): 49–54.

Seaton E.D., Mouser P.E., Charakida A. et al. Investigation of the mechanism of action of nonablative pulsed-dye laser therapy in photorejuvenation and inflammatory acne vulgaris. Br J Dermatol 2006; 155(4): 748–755.

Seeliger S., Buddenkotte J., Schmidt-Choudhury A. et al. Pituitary adenylate cyclase-activating polypeptide: an important vascular regulator in human skin in vivo. Am J Pathol 2010; 177(5): 2563–2575.

Segovia J., Sabbah A., Mgbemena V. et al. TLR2/MyD88/NF-κB pathway, reactive oxygen species, potassium efflux activates NLRP3/ASC inflammasome during respiratory syncytial virus infection. PLoS One 2012; 7(1): 29695.

Seo H.-M., Kim J.-I., Kim H.-S. et al. Prospective comparison of dual wavelength long-pulsed 755-nm Alexandrite/1,064-nm Neodymium:Yttrium-Aluminum-Garnet laser versus 585-nm Pulsed Dye Laser treatment for rosacea. Ann Dermatol 2016; 28(5): 607–614.

Sharquie K.E., Najim R.A., Al-Salman H.N. Oral zinc sulfate in the treatment of rosacea: a double-blind, placebo-controlled study. Int J Dermatol 2006; 45(7): 857–861.

Sheptii O.V. Laser therapy of vascular skin pathology: basic principles and practical recommendations. Apparatnaya kosmetologiya 2018; 1/2: 54–66.

Shi X., Wang L., Li X. et al. Neuropeptides contribute to peripheral nociceptive sensitization by regulating interleukin-1beta production in keratinocytes. Anesth Analg 2011; 113(1): 175–183.

Speeckaert R., Lambert J., Grine L. et al. The many faces of interleukin-17 in inflammatory skin diseases. Br J Dermatol 2016; 175(5): 892–901.

Steinhoff M., Buddenkotte J., Shpacovitch V. et al. Proteinase-activated receptors: transducers of proteinase-mediated signaling in inflammation and immune response. Endocr Rev 2005; 26(1): 1–43.

Storozhuk M.V., Zholos A.V. TRP channels as novel targets for endogenous ligands: focus on endocannabinoids and nociceptive signalling. Curr Neuropharmacol 2018; 16(2): 137–150.

Sulk M., Seeliger S., Aubert J. et al. Distribution and expression of non-neuronal transient receptor potential (TRPV) ion channels in rosacea. J Invest Dermatol 2012; 132(4): 1253–1262.

Tan J., Berg M. Rosacea: current state of epidemiology. J Am Acad Dermatol 2013; 69(6 Suppl 1): 27–35.

Tan J., Steinhoff M., Berg M. et al. Shortcomings in rosacea diagnosis and classification. Br J Dermatol 2017; 176(1): 197–199.

Tsai T.Y., Chiang Y.Y., Huang Y.C. Cardiovascular risk and comorbidities in patients with rosacea: a systematic review and meta-analysis. Acta Derm Venereol. 2020; 100(17): adv00300.

Two A.M., Wu W., Gallo R.L., Hata T.R. Rosacea: Part I. Introduction, categorization, histology, pathogenesis, and risk factors. J Am Acad Dermatol 2015; 72(5): 749–758.

US National Rosacea Society, www rosacea.org.

Urakova D.S., Fominykh E.M. Comparison of different methods of tissue dissection. Plastic Surg Cosmetol 2011; 1: 1–4.

Urakova D.S., Kalashnikova N.G. Spatially modulated ablation (SMA) in the correction of striae. Apparatnaya Kosmetologiya 2015; 3: 58–62.

van der Kolk T., van der Wall H.E.C., Balmforth C. et al. a systematic literature review of the human skin microbiome as biomarker for dermatological drug development. Br J Clin Pharmacol 2018; 84(10): 2178–2193.

Varricchi G., de Paulis A., Marone G., Galli S.J. Future needs in mast cell biology. Int J Mol Sci 2019; 20(18): 4397.

Wang B., Yan B., Zhao Z. et al. Relationship between tea drinking behaviour and rosacea: a clinical case-control study. Acta Derm Venereol 2021; 101(6): adv00488.

Wang L., Wang Y.J., Hao D. et al. The theranostics role of mast cells in the pathophysiology of rosacea. Front Med (Lausanne) 2020; 6: 324.

Wang R., Li R., Wu Y. Skin microbiome in patients with rosacea and healthy controls. E-poster presented at AAD VMX Virtual Meeting Experience 2020, June 12–14.

Wang Y., Zhao Z., Liu F., Xie H. et al. Relationship between the incidence of rosacea and drinking or smoking in China. J Central South University Med Sci. 2020; 45(2): 165–168.

Weinkle A.P., Doktor V., Emer J. Update on the management of rosacea. Clin Cosmet Invest Dermatol 2015; 8: 159–177.

Weiss E., Katta R. Diet and rosacea: the role of dietary change in the management of rosacea. Dermatol Pract Concept 2017; 7(4): 31–37.

Wilkin J., Dahl M., Detmar M. et al. Standard classification system of rosacea: report of the National Rosacea Society Expert Committee on the Classification and Staging of Rosacea. J Am Acad Dermatol 2002; 46: 584–587.

Wohlrab J., Kreft D. Niacinamide — mechanisms of action and its topical use in dermatology. Skin Pharmacol Physiol 2014; 27(6): 311–315.

Woo Y.R., Lim J.H., Cho D.H., Park H.J. Rosacea: molecular mechanisms and management of a chronic cutaneous inflammatory condition. Int J Mol Sci 2016; 17(9): 1562.

Wu C.-Y., Chang Y.-T., Juan C.-K. et al. Risk of inflammatory bowel disease in patients with rosacea: results from a nationwide cohort study in Taiwan. J Am Acad Dermatol 2017; 76(5): 911–917.

Yamasaki K., Gallo R.L., Li G. et al. The molecular pathology of rosacea. J Dermatol Sci 2009; 55(2): 77–81.

Yamasaki K., Kanada K., Macleod D.T. et al. TLR2 expression is increased in rosacea and stimulates enhanced serine protease production by keratinocytes. J Invest Dermatol 2011; 131(3): 688–697.

Yentzer B.A., Fleischer A.B. Jr. Changes in rosacea comorbidities and treatment utilization over time. J Drugs Dermatol 2010; 9(11): 1402–1406.

Yuan C., Ma Y., Wang Y. et al. Rosacea is associated with conjoined interactions between physical barrier of the skin and microorganisms: a pilot study. J Clin Lab Anal 2020; e23363.

Yutskovskaya Y.A., Remenyuk M.G., Naumchik G.A. Clinical experience of botulinum toxin type a application in rosacea therapy. Cosmetics & Medicine 2016; 1: 72–75.

Zhong S., Sun N., Liu X. et al. Topical tranexamic acid improves the permeability barrier in rosacea. Dermatologica Sinica 2015; 33 (2): 112–117.

Zhou L.F., Lu R. Successful treatment of Morbihan disease with total glucosides of paeony: a case report. World J Clin Cases 2022; 10(19): 6688–6694.

Zhou M., Xie H., Cheng L., Li J. Clinical characteristics and epidermal barrier function of papulopustular rosacea: a comparison study with acne vulgaris. Pak J Med Sci 2016; 32(6): 1344–1348.

www.ingramcontent.com/pod-product-compliance
Lightning Source LLC
Chambersburg PA
CBHW052022030426
42335CB00026B/3247